This book is dedicated to
Terri and Spenser Steinman,
and Helen Wisner,
without whose support
this book would not have been possible.

ACKNOWLEDGMENTS

We gratefully acknowledge the help of the following for reviewing all or portions of the manuscript: Ed Begley, Jr.; Russell Blaylock, M.D.; Devra Lee Davis, Ph.D.; Joan Dine; Jay Feldman, National Coalition Against the Misuse of Pesticides; Greenpeace, United States; Jane Hersey, Feingold Association of the United States; Kaye Kilburn, M.D.; Dr. Thomas Lovejoy; Marion Moses, M.D., Pesticide Education Center; Dr. John Olney; Doris Rapp, M.D.; Jeremy Russell; G. Megan Shields, M.D.; Ellen Sibergeld, Ph.D., University of Maryland; Hugh Wilhere; and Brent Wisner.

We also acknowledge the following, whose own research and

writings have provided background: John Adams, Natural Resources Defense Council; Ira Arlook, Sandra Buchanan and Ed Hopkins, Citizen Action; Annie Berthold Bond; John Bower; Lynn Marie Bower; Rachel Carson; Citizens Commission on Human Rights; Theo Colborn, Ph.D.; Samuel S. Epstein, M.D.; Foundation for Advancements in Science and Education; the Honorable Albert Gore; Aubrey Hampton; Denis Hayes; L. Ron Hubbard; William Marcus, Ph.D.; Claudia Miller, M.D.; Ralph Nader; Theron Randolph, M.D.; Dennis Remington, M.D.; H.J. Roberts, M.D.; Janette Sherman, M.D.; Joseph Weissman, M.D.; and Bruce Wiseman.

We also gratefully acknowledge the help of the following, who have acted decisively on their similar concerns: Kirstie Alley and Parker Stevenson; Senator Barbara Boxer; Glenn Braswell; Senator Patrick Leahy; Alex Schauss, Ph.D.; John Travolta and Kelly Preston; and Tom Cruise and Nicole Kidman.

We wish to thank Terry Zeyen and Robert Basile for their research assistance; Sheila M. Curry for her excellent editing, and our literary agent, Madeleine Morel, for helping to bring this project from concept to reality.

LIVING HEALTHY
in a TOXIC WORLD

LIVING HEALTHY
in a TOXIC WORLD

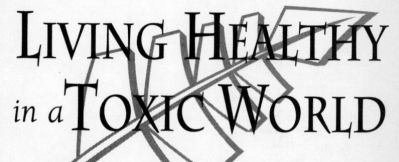

*Simple Steps to Protect You and Your Family
From Everyday Chemicals, Poisons, and Pollution*

DAVID STEINMAN

and

R. MICHAEL WISNER

A Perigee Book

A Perigee Book
Published by The Berkley Publishing Group
200 Madison Avenue
New York, NY 10016

Copyright © 1996 by David Steinman and Michael Wisner
Book design by Irving Perkins Associates
Cover design Dale Fiorillo

First edition: August 1996

Published simultaneously in Canada.

The Putnam Berkley World Wide Web site address is
http://www.berkley.com

Library of Congress Cataloging-in-Publication Data

Steinman, David.
    Living healthy in a toxic world : simple steps to protect you and
  your family from everyday chemicals, poison, and pollution / by
  David Steinman and R. Michael Wisner ; foreword by Kirstie Alley.—
  1st ed.
        p. cm.
    Includes bibliographical references.
    ISBN 0-399-52206-9
    1. Toxicology—Popular works.   2. Health.   I. Wisner, R. Michael.
  II. Title.
  RA1213.S72   1996
  615.9—dc20   95-43241
                                                                   CIP

Printed in the United States of America

10   9   8   7   6   5   4   3   2

CONTENTS

FOREWORD

I was sitting in a doctor's office, probably the tenth doctor I had seen in the last year. I had had about every test in the book and every orifice of my body poked and explored. Although that felt good, I was still sick. I'd been X-rayed, CAT scanned, MRI'd, and who knows what else. I was tired. I was always tired. I had these weird nervous tremors, dizziness, and a pain in my neck so severe I wanted to scream. It was nearly impossible to work. The doctor looked at me like I was a Vulcan. I told him that was only a movie. He said all my tests were negative, and there was no reason for me to feel like a person on the verge of dying. He suggested I see a psychiatrist he knew. I politely told him to get screwed; I'd been nuts my whole life, but only sick for the last two years. Then I left.

I felt as helpless as if I was gasping for my last breath. I decided that the one thing I could possibly do was to change my diet, and that maybe would make me feel a little better.

I went to see an M.D. named Megan Shields for a nutritional program. Her administrator asked me, out of nowhere, if I had experienced a major environmental change before I got sick. I had. My husband and I had moved into our new home. We called it the "death house" because both of us had been sick ever since. He said, "Your house was tented and gassed for termites before you moved in." How the heck did he know that? He pulled one of those thick books about chemicals off a shelf and showed me the symptoms of methyl bromide exposure. I had nine of the ten symptoms. I called my realtor. Yep, they had used the stuff to gas the termites. But "it was perfectly safe." Right, and Mussolini was cool. Anyway, my doctor's exam and tests confirmed the methyl bromide was the cause of my problems. Fortunately, I went through the detoxification program in this book and was fine. But I was ticked off. How many of my friends were being poisoned in their homes without knowing it? How many people with a chemical exposure get misdiagnosed by a doctor every day?

Awake and eating well, I started looking around my home. Pet chemicals, garden sprays, pesticides, herbicides, cans of cleaning stuff, paints, and glues. I had dreams of Greenpeacers chained to my front door with a banner reading, "Stop Toxic Waste Dumping Now," while two wild-eyed shrinks carted me away for more tests. I met with the Natural Resources Defense Council and Meryl Streep, who was working with them, and learned how many deadly chemicals were sprayed on the food I was eating. I figured I'd stop acting, become anorexic, and start modeling jeans. I had to find people who knew what was safe and what wasn't. Where the hell were all the experts? I *liked* my life; I was not about to move to a mountaintop and start rubbing sticks together and eating berries.

Then Nirvana struck. The two guys who wrote this book knew more and had more practical solutions than any of the hundreds of people I harassed for answers. Their book ingeniously blends a sense of humor with simple, everyday things you can do to protect your health. It makes it easy and entertaining to do things that can make profound improvements in the quality of your life.

As a mother with two spectacular children, I use this book daily. It has made an enormous difference in our lives. Everyone's happier, brighter, and healthier. It's good for the environment and saves me money too. The way I see it, no one can lose. So buy it, read it, use it, then be sure and memorize it—that way you can recycle it for toilet paper or kindling. Have fun.

Love,
Kirstie Alley

INTRODUCTION

1. ALL YOU EVER NEEDED TO KNOW ABOUT TOXIC CHEMICALS BUT GOVERNMENT AND INDUSTRY WOULD NEVER TELL YOU

"The greatest danger of pollution may well be that we shall tolerate levels of it so low as to have no acute nuisance value, but sufficiently high, nevertheless, to cause delayed disease and spoil the quality of life."

—RENE DUBOIS,
Environmentalist/Scientist (1968)

Do horror movies scare the pants off you? Do you drop your Good & Plenty just at the scariest part? When you see a news report preaching nothing but doom and gloom, do you instantly start channel surfing? While the health impact of toxic chemicals is a real horror story, you can't just drop your candy or surf. The health of you and your family is too important. We are going to spell out clear and present environmental health risks, while at the same time maintaining a sense of humor and providing you with steps you can take that will have a positive effect on your health.

Just the Facts, Ma'am, Just the Facts . . .

Many chemicals and their residues build up in the body's tissues. Others do immediate damage and disappear, leaving no trace whatsoever. There have been more than four million distinct chemical compounds identified since 1965, with nearly six thousand new compounds being added to the list each week nowadays. Few have been tested for all their health effects. We now use more than fifty thousand chemicals in daily living; more than three thousand chemicals are deliberately added to food. More than seven hundred chemicals have been identified in drinking water alone. The United States Environmental Protection Agency (EPA) has reported nearly thirty cancer-causing chemicals detectable in the fat tissues of literally every American today. The average home contains more than one thousand different chemicals. Chemicals are a part of every aspect of our daily life, from the grocery store to our child's nursery to the kitchen tap. These facts are undisputed. It's time to take the gloves off (or maybe put them back on) and get to work.

The potential ill effects from many of these chemicals are not known, but there is overwhelming scientific evidence showing that many chemicals previously thought safe are not, and that we have been deceived by both industry and government. We now know that very low levels of some common chemicals cause harm. We now know that the immune and nervous systems are also targets. For you or your children this might translate into lowered IQ, allergies, reduced resistance to the common cold, sexual problems, memory loss, and more—in short, a real attack on the very quality of our daily lives.

The worst harm is to our children, whose small bodies and underdeveloped immune systems can't always effectively cope with today's chemicals. Some scientists working for industry will tell you cancer is decreasing or held in check or just hitting us more because we live longer. In fact, one of the most rapidly increasing rates of cancer is in children under the age of thirteen.

The consequences of industrial pollution touch everyone, piercing all racial, economic, and political boundaries. Studies have shown urban children have IQs several points lower than average just from the quantity of lead in their environment. A major study of a metropolitan area showed sixteen hundred premature deaths from air pollution each year. If clean air laws were simply complied with, the health savings would amount to billions of dollars. The Russians have asked American scientists for assistance in detoxifying their workforce, which has been exposed to toxins without protection for years. Now these workers have to compete in a free marketplace, their productivity seriously damaged by toxic chemicals. In the United States, experts fear that increased crime, education failures, loss of productivity, and skyrocketing health care costs are due, in part, to pollution. We are coming to the powerful realization that environmental responsibility is ultimately in both our best health *and* economic interests.

Before radio talk show hosts go berserk and denounce this little book with screams of "environmental scare tactics," realize the very values they hold so dear—intelligence, responsibility for self, education, family, reduced costs of doing business, indeed our very ability to compete in an international market—are also equally threatened. Taking care of your health is a smart thing. It's easy. You don't have to be a member of one political party or another.

Super health, all around—it's good for body, mind, and soul. We're going to show you simple things you can do that will improve your health, bring you a greater feeling of well-being, and maybe even begin to ease the cloud of pollution that threatens the planet we all share. We're going to show you simple things you can do that could save your life.

2. IF YOU DON'T KNOW THE WORDS, YOU

CAN'T SING THE TUNE

Nearly thirty million Americans are functionally illiterate.

It happens all the time. You flip on your car radio, or your TV at home, and someone is talking about the "environment" or "health." Whether they are experts or consumer advocates, they spend most of the time arguing with another expert. The subject's important, so you listen up. Then it happens. The fifty-cent words start flying around like darts that would pierce a *Webster's* dictionary. What are these guys talking about? "Heavy metals." Right. Isn't that some kind of rock-and-roll music? "Reaction time." That's how long it takes Harry to make it from the bathroom to the couch at halftime. Anyway, you're bored now and start looking for the chips and dip. Or, while driving, you might make a profane gesture at the guy who just cut you off, only to realize it's your boss. Later, your mind wanders back to the show. Did anyone understand them, or are you just dumb? Don't worry; you're not alone.

Have you ever read one of those manuals on how to program your VCR, and quit before you were finished because of too many terms and words you didn't understand? Would you want a mechanic working on your car or a doctor working on you if they didn't understand their training manuals? The result might be worse than what you did to that VCR.

Whether it's hitting a baseball, fixing an engine, or understanding the environment or the human body, you have to understand the basic words in order to be successful. If you do, something that looks complex gets easy—fast.

But some people might not want it that simple. So they sit in an ivory tower charging three hundred dollars an hour to explain technical terms. They want to make the subject appear complex. They want to intimidate you. It's nonsense. A major corporate executive hired two Ph.D.'s to explain technical environmental terms and concepts. He could have saved the company money, and himself some intellectual honesty, by getting a good environmental dictionary.

In this day and age when TV's "talking heads" bend and mangle the truth for their own agendas, it is hard to understand what is true and who is right about the environment or about health issues. Is cancer really on the rise? Is pollution affecting our health, shortening our lives? Should we be concerned about pesticides in our food, in our homes? The real answers to these and other important questions can only be determined by you. You have to sift through the information, understand it, and make up your own mind, come to your own conclusions. This is judgment. This is intelligence. You have to understand the words. Then you can understand, decide, and act. Then you can contribute. In the back of this book you will find the most commonly used environmental and health words defined. You should turn to that section and read these before going on.

SIMPLE THINGS TO DO

- Always use a good dictionary to define any word or term you don't fully understand.
- Review the words and terms in the Glossary in the back of this book.

RESOURCES

Toxics A to Z: A Guide to Everyday Pollution Hazards

A compilation of a wide range of environmental health issues and terms in simple language, by John Harte and others (University of California Press, Berkeley and Los Angeles, 1991).

Cry Out: An Illustrated Guide to What You Can Do to Save the Earth

For a free booklet with an illustrated glossary of environmental terms for children: The Alley Foundation, P.O. Box 5769, Beverly Hills CA 90209.

3. EVERYBODY'S TALKIN'

Our Fair Sister

"As each one of you stands alone in God's knowledge, so must each one of you be alone in his knowledge of God and his understanding of the earth."

—KAHLIL GIBRAN,
The Prophet

Precious Planet

"The question is whether any civilization can wage relentless war on life without destroying itself, and without losing the right to be called civilized."

—RACHEL CARSON,
Silent Spring

"The environment we have created may now be a major cause of death in the U.S. Cancer, heart disease, and lung disease, accounting for 12 percent of deaths in 1900 and 38 percent in 1940, were the cause of 59 percent of all deaths in 1976. . . . Growing evidence links much of the occurrence of these diseases . . . to the nature of the environment."

—MICHAEL J. CANLON,
*EPA Cites U.S. Environment as a
Leading Cause of Death*

"Several government reports . . . conclude that 60 to 90 percent of all types of cancers in the U.S. are causally related to environmental factors ranging from food preservatives and additives to toxic chemical substances."

—Douglas M. Costle,
Administrator of the United States
Environmental Protection Agency,
*Defense by Disaster: Proving the
Value of Environmental Protection*

So Sweet

"Experimental animals given artificial sweetener in their drinking water ate more and became fatter. Only when the artificial sweetener was given in massive enough dosages to make the food taste bad did the animals eat less over the long run."

—Dennis Remington, M.D.,
*The Bitter Truth About Artificial
Sweeteners*

The Paycheck

"It can be calculated that approximately 50,000 to 70,000 deaths and 350,000 new cases of illness each year in this country are caused by toxic occupational exposure."

—Philip J. Landrigan, M.D.,
"Current Status of Occupational
Disease in the United States,"
*Journal of Occupational Medicine
and Toxicology*

Blowing in the Wind

"A study commissioned by the U.S. EPA concluded that wages lost by American workers suffering from just air pollution alone total a whopping $36 billion a year."

—Douglas M. Costle,
Administrator of the United States
Environmental Protection Agency,
*Defense by Disaster: Proving the
Value of Environmental Protection*

"The Office of Technology Assessment says that air pollution may cause 50,000 premature deaths in the U.S. every year."

—U.S. Congress, Office of
Technology Assessment, *Acid Rain
and Transported Air Pollutants:
Implications for Public Policy*

The Poison Within

"We are exposed to an overwhelming number of chemical contaminants every day in our air, water, food, and general environment. . . . Many industrial and agricultural compounds were specifically formulated to resist the decompositional effects of heat, abrasion, water, and chemical agents. . . . Many chemicals tend to accumulate in the body's fat tissues, where they may persist indefinitely. This process is called toxic bioaccumulation. A national survey by the U.S. EPA found most Americans have dozens of identifiable contaminants in their fatty tissue."

—THERON G. RANDOLPH, M.D.,
An Alternative Approach to Allergies

"The fact that the suburbanite is not instantly stricken has little meaning, for the toxins may sleep long in his body, to become manifest months or years later in an obscure disorder almost impossible to trace to its origins."

—RACHEL CARSON,
Silent Spring

Drugs

"According to a detailed study published by a Senate subcommittee in 1962, of the 4,000 drug products legally marketed in the country over the previous 24 years, almost half had no scientifically proven value and little has changed since that time."

—JEREMY RIFKIN,
Entropy into the Greenhouse World

"Adverse drug effects now rank among the top 10 causes of hospitalization and are held accountable for as many as 50 million hospital patient days a year."

—MILTON SILVERMAN and
PHILIP LEE, *Pills, Profits and Politics*

Small World

"NRDC estimates that at least 17 percent of the preschool population, or three million children, receive exposure to neurotoxic organophosphate insecticides, just from *raw* fruits and vegetables, that are above levels the federal government considers safe. High level exposure to these insecticides can cause nausea, convulsions, coma, and even death. Dietary exposure may [cause] behavioral impairments and alter neurological function."

—NATURAL RESOURCE DEFENSE
COUNCIL, *Intolerable Risk:*
Pesticides in Our Children's Food

Take Your Vitamins

"Fatalities Resulting from Poisonings by Vitamin Supplements in the United States

1987:	0	1989:	0
1988:	0	1990:	1

"Fatalities Resulting from All Major Categories of Prescription and Non-Prescription Pharmaceutical Drugs (not including illegal drugs)

1987:	325	1989:	453
1988:	434	1990:	487"

—"WHICH IS SAFER: DRUGS OR
VITAMINS?"
Townsend Letter for Doctors

More Isn't Better

"Since the 1940s pesticide use has increased tenfold, but crop losses to insects have doubled."

—NATURAL RESOURCES DEFENSE
COUNCIL, *Intolerable Risk:
Pesticides in Our Children's Food*

Part I

HOME, HONEY

--- ✿ ---

4. CLEAN HOUSE

"Like all occupations, housework has its hazards. . . . Perhaps the most serious exposure is to modern household cleaners which may contain a number of proven and suspect causes of cancer."

—DAVID STERLING, Ph.D.,
Old Dominion University[1]

When Harry Found Sally

When Harry gets home from work at the Air Quality Management District, he can't help noticing how the windows shine, the counters sparkle, the kitchen glistens, and the bathroom is spotless. He is very proud of the beautiful home Sally has made for the family. But where *is* Sally? He finds her in the bedroom lying on the bed in a comatose state, clutching a bottle of furniture polish, babbling to herself about Leona Helmsley biting Brad Pitt's neck.

BACKGROUND

Here you are trying to make your home safer and healthier. You pull out the cleanser and start scouring the sink. But what you don't know is that one of the ingredients in your favorite brand could be a highly abrasive powder, crystalline silica, that causes cancer and scars the lungs.[2]

Or you may suddenly learn that your furniture polish, the one you've been using for years, is being pulled off the market because it contains cancer-causing formaldehyde.

There are no warnings on labels about any of this. No safety guidelines on the package. No hint of danger in those catchy commercials, no fine print in the ads.

Although the Food and Drug Administration won't admit it, the EPA denies it, and the federal Consumer Product Safety Commission (CPSC) downplays it . . .

Your health is under siege by toxic invaders that you bring home from the market every time you shop.

DID YOU KNOW:

- Fifty-two thousand household product-related hospital emergency room admissions were reported in 1990.[3]
- Excess cancer deaths occur among homemakers when compared to women who work outside the home.[4]
- "The excess prevalence of cancers among homemakers relative to employed women may be due to the occupational exposures of homemaking . . ."[5]
- Although two leading brands of household cleanser, Ajax and Zud, contain crystalline silica, neither Congress nor the CPSC has proposed laws or regulations to require label disclosure of these or virtually any other cancer-causing chemicals found in household products.[6]
- One of the most common chemicals found in household cleaning products is butyl cellosolve, which is toxic to the blood cells, kidneys, and liver.[7] It is absorbed through the skin.[8] The nation's

most popular brand of window cleaner, Windex, contains butyl cellosolve, but it's not on the label.[9,10] This stuff can do a lot more (to you) than just clean your windows.

- A toxic chemical, dichlorobenzene, used widely in room deodorizers and moth repellents, has been found in the blood of over ninety-five percent of children and adults tested throughout the country.[11]
- Many other chemicals in household cleaning products, including those that cause cancer, nerve damage, and birth defects, are also absorbed through the skin.[12]
- The New York Poison Control Center reported that eighty-five percent of product warning labels are inadequate.[13]
- Every year there are between five and ten million household poisonings.[14]
- Federally required warning labels are required **only** on products that are **immediately** harmful or fatal if swallowed or inhaled—not something many of us do every day. No warnings are required on products that can affect your health over time. But isn't that the way most of us use household products—over time?
- *Inert* on a product label does NOT mean *inert*. Of the fourteen hundred chemicals the EPA allows industry to list as "inert ingredients," forty are known to cause cancer, brain damage, or other chronic effects; another sixty-four are classed as potentially toxic.[15]

SIMPLE THINGS TO DO

Prepare your own safe, effective homemade cleaners. Three we recommend:

- *All-around cleanser:* Mix 3 teaspoons of borax, 4 tablespoons of distilled white vinegar, and 2 cups of hot water (so borax will dissolve) together in a refillable spray bottle. Shake well. You can use this mix to clean just about any kind of light mess. It is best when used warm.
- *Cleaning up grease:* Add ½ to 1 teaspoon washing soda (also

known as sodium carbonate, soda ash, or sal soda) and ¼ to 1 teaspoon liquid soap, if you need something stronger.

• *Bleaching:* Use hydrogen peroxide or sodium perborate instead of chlorine bleach. They're safer.
• *Wood furniture polish:* Mix ½ teaspoon of walnut or olive oil and ¼ cup of vinegar. Cover when storing.
• *All-purpose floor cleaner:* Mix ¼ cup liquid soap and ¼ cup lemon juice in 2 gallons of warm water.
• *Natural disinfectant:* Mix 2 tablespoons Australian tea tree oil with 2 cups of water in spray bottle.

Follow these tips when using homemade recipes:

• *For a light and airy fragrance:* Add a few drops of your favorite essential oil to the above recipes. Essential oils are available at health food stores.
• *For enhanced abrasion:* Use a Scotch-Brite Soft Scour No-Scratch sponge.

Grandma's Pantry

20 Mule Team Borax, distilled white vinegar, washing soda, hydrogen peroxide, and sodium perborate can be purchased at health food stores, drugstores, and some supermarkets. Virtually all supermarkets and health stores carry 20 Mule Team Borax and distilled white vinegar. Arm & Hammer is a good brand of washing soda. If your store does not carry washing soda, call Arm & Hammer at (800) 524-1328. If your store does not carry sodium perborate, call a local chemical supply company (see your Yellow Pages). Any supermarket brand of distilled white vinegar will work fine. A small funnel helps when filling spray bottles.

Product	The Problem	The Solution
Aerosols	Toxic to brain and heart.	Don't use. Use a pump sprayer or apply by hand.

Product	The Problem	The Solution
Oven Cleaner	Harmful to eyes and lungs.	Self-cleaning oven. Paste of baking soda and hot water with steel wool.
Furniture/Floor Polish	Causes weakness, sweating, fatigue, headache, depression. Damages liver, brain, and kidney.[16]	Dust with damp cloth. Plain mineral or vegetable oil with vitamin E as a preservative.
Window Cleaners	Poison. Irritant to eyes and lungs.	Nontoxic commercial window cleaner, or mix half water, half white vinegar in pump spray.
Disinfectants	Damage brain. Nausea, weakness, dizziness, chest pains, and skin problems. Cancer.[17]	Air and light. Hot water and borax.
Metal Polish	Burns eyes and skin.[18]	Silver: baking soda, salt, and water. Brass: salt, flour, and vinegar. Copper: lemon juice and salt. Chrome: rubbing alcohol. Aluminum: lemon juice.
Mothballs	Toxic to brain, liver, and blood. Stores in body. Inhaled. Children mistake for candy.[19]	Cedar blocks and chips. Bags of lavender, cloves, rosemary, and lemon peels.

Product	The Problem	The Solution
Drain Cleaners	Burn tissue and eyes. Can explode.	Metal drain snake. Drain baskets. One cup of baking soda followed by one half cup of vinegar. Let sit and flush with hot water.
Air Fresheners	Damage liver, kidney, and brain. Cancer. Builds up in body.[20]	Plants. Fresh flowers. Open windows.
Pesticides		See Chapter 10.
Paint Products		See Chapter 7.

5. Pull the Rug Out

"Carpeting has been shown to contain as many as 10,000,000 organisms per square foot."

—Roger L. Anderson[1]

Synthetic carpeting. It's a relic of better living through chemistry. It came as a *gift* from chemical companies in the 1950s and ever since the American home has never been the same. It's Rob and Laura Petrie and shag carpeting in the "burbs." Like the "burbs" themselves, carpets are the perfect trap. They trap lead, dirt, fleas, and dust mites that crawl up your nose, dog and cat hairs you inhale, and many other noxious substances. What's growing in there, anyway? Is this where you and your kids want to eat your snacks?

Whatever happened to the good ol' hardwood floor? It's healthy. It's clean. It isn't a filter or growing bed for every thing you track in. If you want to get the dust out, it helps to get out the carpet.

Call These on the Carpet

4-phenylcyclohexane (4 PC): A residue in carpet latex backing associated with dizziness, headaches, blurred vision, skin problems, and breathing difficulty.[2]

Isocyanate: A chemical used in carpet glues that damages the brain, nervous system, skin, and lungs.[3]

Styrene: A chemical used in manufacturing carpet that can be inhaled and damages the nervous system, as well as causing irritation of the nose, mouth, and lungs.[4]

DID YOU KNOW:

- Until the 1950s most carpeting was made from natural fibers such as cotton or wool. These days carpeting is produced from a witches' brew of chemical toxins that can contaminate your home's air.[5] New wall-to-wall carpets are covered with a synthetic backing that can expose you to toxic chemical gases.[6]
- Many brands of carpets are treated with moth repellents, mold retardants, and pesticides, all of which poison both the bugs and *you*.
- Toluene, xylene, and styrene are nerve toxins found in carpeting. Not surprisingly, our tissues are also contaminated with these toxins.
- Common symptoms reported by people suffering from toxic carpet exposures include: difficulty breathing, burning eyes, headaches, nausea, rashes, and various illnesses from a weakened immune system.[7]
- One of your worst exposures to lead can come from carpeting. We track in street dirt containing lead. It builds up in the carpet. You could sell mineral rights to your family room!
- Most conventional vacuum cleaners pick up large dirt particles

but spit smaller ones out the exhaust. Take a damp handkerchief and place it over the exhaust while you vacuum. Look at it. That's what you're breathing while you're "cleaning."[8]

- Kawasaki syndrome, an illness causing high fever, is increasingly observed in children after carpet cleaning. Many experts suspect a toxic or infectious agent becomes airborne during carpet cleaning.[9]

- One study found cancer-causing chemicals in every carpet tested.[10]

A Story That Will Floor You

A family had new carpeting installed in their New England home. Within days the parents and five children were inexplicably ill. The mother, remembering that the carpet installers were sick during the installation, asked her family doctor if the new carpet could be the culprit. He didn't know. She discovered the carpeting with latex backing had been rushed from the factory and not properly cured. She saved samples. After being told she was crazy or worse, she finally found Anderson Laboratories. The laboratory does tests in which mice are exposed to carpet samples and observed for health effects. When they were exposed to her samples, the mice died. After the family lost their home, fought lawsuits, testified before Congress, and underwent a successful detoxification treatment (see Chapter 20), their lives were saved, but they'll never be the same.

SIMPLE THINGS TO DO

- Replace your carpeting with hardwood floors. Use nontoxic glues, varnishes, stains, and sealers.
- Use linoleum made from all natural materials (not "synthetic linoleum," which contains chemicals). It comes in a variety of colors and is made from all natural materials.
- Ceramic tile adds beauty to a home and is a wise choice over carpet. Install it with a nontoxic cement adhesive.

- Use natural fiber wool and cotton throw rugs.
- Don't track in the lead and dirt. Leave your shoes at the door.
- If you purchase new carpet, buy natural wool or cotton without chemical additives and latex backings. Use nontoxic padding.
- Make sure new carpet has a certification label stating that the chemical emissions fall below industry standards. This label, however, does not apply to padding or adhesives; toxic emissions still might affect sensitive people.
- Don't use industrial glues to install. Good ol' Elmer's will do fine.
- When new carpet is installed, leave the room and allow the area to fully air out for at least a day. Renting an industrial cleaner and steam cleaning new carpets with hot water ONLY will remove some residual chemicals.
- Apply a carpet sealer, which provides a protective coating, thereby reducing what you breathe.
- Don't use industrial cleaners or spot removers. These contain highly toxic ingredients. Liquid natural soap in a carpet steam cleaner will do just fine.
- Use a vacuum that won't exhaust toxins into your home.

RESOURCES

Nontoxic Carpet and Padding

Hendericksen Naturlich Flooring and Interiors

7120 Keating Avenue
Sebastopol CA 95472
(707)829-3959

Flowright International Products

1495 N.W. Gilman Blvd., #4
Issaquah WA 98027
(206)392-8357

Nature's Carpet
Environmental Home Center
(206)682-7332

World Fibre
P.O. Box 480805
Denver CO 80248
(303)628-2210

Foreign Accents
2825 E. Broadbent Parkway N. E.
Albuquerque, NM 87107
(505)344-4833

Natural Linoleum

Forbo North America
P.O. Box 667
Hazelton PA 18201
(800)459-0771

Non Toxic Environments
9392 S. Gribble Road
Canby OR 97013
(503)266-5244

Carpet Sealants and Nontoxic Adhesives

AMF
1960 Chicago Avenue, Suite E7
Riverside CA 92507
(909)781-6860

Nontoxic Vacuums

Amway
(800)269-2928

Nilfisk
(610)647-6420

Aquamate
(800)225-3878

Networking

Toxic Carpet Information Exchange
P.O. Box 39344
Cincinnati OH 45239

A consumer information clearinghouse for carpet hazards

Consumer Product Safety Commission
Carpet Complaints, Room 529
U.S. Consumer Product Safety Commission
Washington DC 20207
Toll-free hotline: (800)638-2772

6. WHAT'S THAT DIRTY, GAUZY THING IN MY FURNACE?

"Sufficient evidence exists to conclude that indoor air pollution represents a major portion of the public's exposure to air pollution and may pose serious acute and chronic health risks."

—EPA

Once every year or so you wander down to that dark, murky place in the jungle you call your basement and inspect your home's heating and air conditioning unit. It's like a scene from *Tales From the Crypt* as you cautiously trudge through the darkness, expecting spiders to drop on your head any moment! You pry open the unit to find this horrible dirty, gauzy thing stuffed full of dirt and slime. It's yucky, and, when you start to pull it out, little green things start scrambling up your arm. You heave it. It's alive. You're so grossed out that you dart to the nearest phone and call around looking for the producers of *Outbreak* so you can borrow one of those suits Dustin Hoffman wore. Maybe you just leave it. What does all this have to do with your health, anyway? A lot! Many toxins get into your body because of something you do every moment of every day: breathe.

DID YOU KNOW:

- Your cooling and heating unit, if not cleaned regularly and filtered, circulates asbestos, pesticides, cleaning chemicals, tobacco smoke, rat feces, dust mites, bacteria, cooking gases, and radon. These are associated with headaches, fatigue, allergies, eye, skin and lung irritation, cancer, nerve damage, and birth defects.[1,2,3,4,5,6]
- The EPA reports that eight of the most common indoor pollutants cost the nation more than one billion dollars a year in medical costs from cancer and heart disease alone.[7]

SIMPLE THINGS TO DO

- Electrostatic filters, relying on the principle of static electricity, collect pollution particles. They go in where that dirty, gauzy thing went. They filter more pollution than that dirty, gauzy thing, including molds, bacteria, and smoke. They're washable, reusable, and pay for themselves within a short time.
- When was the last time you had your air ducts and vents cleaned? What's growing in there? Inexpensive services will come to your home and fully clean ducts and vents. Don't let them use toxic cleaners or disinfectants. Just have them cleaned with simple nontoxic supplies (see Chapter 4).
- Check the area where your unit draws air. Often it's near, or in, a dusty closet, basement, laundry room, or garage. Clear out all old paints, rags, and sources of chemicals or dust.
- If your unit's intake is in a garage, keep the door open—more fresh air.
- Keep your home's doors and windows open as much as possible.

RESOURCES

Electrostatic Filters

AllerMed Corp
31 Steel Road
Wiley TX 75098
(214)442-4898

Nigra Enterprises
5699 Kanan Road
Agoura CA 91301
(818)889-6877

Ozark Water Service and Environmental Services
114 Spring St.
Sulphur Springs AR 72768
(800)835-8908

7. PAINT YOUR WAGON

"100 painters were randomly selected and tested. Almost without exception, they had measurable amounts of toxic chemicals from paints stored in their bodies. Chemicals were found in their blood, fat, even hair. Nearly one third were suffering from health problems."

—D. L. CURTIS, M.D.[1]

Mark Twain Revisited . . .

Defense Attorney: Objection, your honor.

The Judge: Overruled. Answer the question, Mr. Sawyer.

Tom Sawyer: I wuz jus tired.

Plaintiff Attorney: You were just tired, Mr. Sawyer, so you conned Mr. Finn into painting Aunt Sally's fence for nothing?

Tom Sawyer: Not fur nuthin. I wuz gonna pay 'im.

Plaintiff Attorney: Pay him what, Mr. Sawyer?

Tom Sawyer: Three slim jims, they wuz good, too.

Plaintiff Attorney: Three slim jims, Mr. Sawyer? You wouldn't part with three slim jims. What was your real reason, Mr. Sawyer? Answer the question.

Defense Attorney: Objection, your honor; he's badgering the witness.

The Judge: Overruled, counselor. Answer the question, Mr. Sawyer.

Tom Sawyer: Well, ya see . . .

Plaintiff Attorney: See what, Mr. Sawyer?

Tom Sawyer: Well, me an Jim, we'd gonna go down the river cuz that stuff give me a hedache.

Plaintiff Attorney: So you had my client paint the fence for you?

Tom Sawyer: Yes'im.

Plaintiff Attorney: Well, Mr. Sawyer, my client has a six-million-dollar law suit against you for personal injuries sustained as a consequence of painting Aunt Sally's fence. He is disabled in the hospital with seizures, headaches, and freckles that are falling off his face. What do you have to say about that, Mr. Sawyer?

Tom Sawyer: I'll pay 'im the three slim jims?

Maybe Tom Sawyer knew what he was doing when he conned Huck Finn into painting Aunt Sally's fence. On the other hand, the seventy-five percent of Americans who paint their own homes probably don't know what they're doing (to their health).[2] What's more, it's no longer just painting: It's sanding, stripping, undercoating, varnishing, spraying, glazing, staining, sealing. Each of these activities can expose you to toxic chemicals. Each of these can affect your health.

DID YOU KNOW:

- Chemicals in paint products enter your body through the skin, eyes, and respiratory passages. They can cause eye, skin, and lung irritation, lowered sperm count, damaged kidneys, high blood pressure, headaches, birth defects, cancer, brain damage, and more.[3]
- Commercial paint contains nerve toxins and cancer-causing chemicals including formaldehyde, methylene chloride, xylene, and toluene, and a host of others.[4,5]
- The federal government reports that over ninety percent of all Americans have measurable amounts of toluene, xylene, styrene, benzene, and ethylbenzene stored in their bodies.[6] These are chemicals found in everyday paint products.[7] Brings a whole new meaning to *body paint.*
- People who paint are at high risk for allergies and severe skin rashes.[8]
- Painters have a forty-percent higher rate of cancer than the population's average. Their children have higher than average rates of leukemia.[9]
- Families with painters have higher rates of birth defects.[10]

Take It Off, Take It All Off!

The largest source of lead exposure is from the old paint on walls peeling and flaking into dust. Many paints manufactured before 1975 contain lead. If you sand or burn this old paint, you are breathing lead. A coat of nontoxic paint and sealer will provide protection. Removing lead paint by sanding or burning can increase the lead dust in homes one hundred to one thousand times.[11] You'd be safer sitting on a smokestack. If you decide to remove all old lead paint, consult a professional.

Are Artists Naturally Crazy or Just Toxic?

Van Gogh was said to pick his nails clean with his teeth. He went nuts. Toxic nuts? Artists work closely with their materials and often take few precautions. The brain toxins mercury and lead are present in many pigments along with other toxins including cadmium, cobalt, and arsenic. Paints, varnishes, and cleaning materials contain benzene and other solvents that are toxic to brain cells. Screen painting uses toxic dyes and benzene solutions. A review of the ingredient list for Grumbacher Paints (a popular brand for artists) shows they contain PCBs, hexachlorobenzene, and many other toxic substances. Sometimes what glitters is more than gold. It's cadmium, chromium, and cobalt too!

SIMPLE THINGS TO DO

- Use latex (water-based) or other least toxic brands of paints indoors.
- Open all the windows. Ventilation. Ventilation. Ventilation.
- For extra protection, purchase a respirator that covers your mouth and nose. Always wear a dust mask or respirator when sanding wood.
- Wear nonpermeable gloves.
- Always store toxic paint products safely in airtight containers, away from living areas. AN ARTIST WHO PAINTS AND SLEEPS IN HIS LOFT WILL PROBABLY DIE IN HIS LOFT.
- Use a nontoxic sealer that locks in fumes so you don't breathe them.
- Avoid paint strippers listing methylene chloride as an ingredient. Use nontoxic brands.
- Don't sand or burn off old paint.

RESOURCES

Paint Products

AFM Enterprises

1140 Stacy Court
Riverside CA 92507
(909)781-6860

Homestead Paint and Finishes

P.O. Box 1668
Lunenburg MA 01462
(508)582-6426

Klean Strip

P.O. Box 1879
Memphis TN 38101
(901)775-0100

Livos Company

614 Agua Fria St.
Santa Fe NM 87501
(505)988-9111

Miller Paint Company

317 S.E. Grand Avenue
Portland OR 97214
(503)233-4491

Safety Equipment

Orr Safety Equipment

P.O. Box 16326
Louisville KY 40256
(800)726-6789

Artistic Painting Safety

Center for Safety in the Arts
5 Beekman Street, Suite 820
New York NY 10038
(212)227-6220

Others

Environmental Hazards Management Institute
10 Newmarket Rd.
P.O. Box 932
Durham NH 03824
(603)868-1496

8. WIRED!

"No fewer than twelve childhood and occupational studies—all of them conducted, published, or re-analyzed between 1985 and 1989—showed significantly increased rates of brain cancer among people exposed to electromagnetic fields at home and at work."

—*The Great Power Line Cover-Up*[1]

Mildred and Priscilla are driving down the road on a sweltering Midwestern afternoon in their 1972 beige sedan. Each proudly sports a new bouffant hairdo because it is Saturday and they have hot dates. Off to the side of the road stretches a chain of towering metal high-tension poles. As they near the poles, both Mildred and Priscilla's hair goes ballistic and starts to rise. Within seconds they look like they just plugged their newly manicured nails into two-twenty electric sockets. Mildred screams as she tries to unglue her hair—plastered to the ceiling of the car, "This humidity is ruining my hair!" It's not the humidity, Mildred. . . .

Enough to Make Your Hair Stand on End . . .

TVs, high tension wires, computer terminals, radios, hair dryers, and microwave ovens all give off electromagnetic radiation and form electromagnetic fields (EMFs).

These fields pose health risks.[2,3,4]

EMFs are measured by gauss units (a measurement of magnetic fields named after German mathematician K.F. Gauss). A milligauss (mG) is equal to a thousandth of a gauss. Many scientists feel that a level of less than three mG is safe. However, a growing number of scientists feel a safe level is less than one mG.[5] Let's look at your home:

Source of EMFs in Home[6,7]	Gauss Reading (mG)
Refrigerator (depending on model/age)	2 to 16
Hair dryer	100
Electric shaver	100
Television/computer monitor	7
Electric blanket (pre-1987)	10
Microwave oven	37
Radiant heating (floor, ceiling, baseboard)	27
Fluorescent light fixtures	6
High-tension wires (100–500 feet away)	5
Improperly grounded wiring	5 or more

The Three D's: Degree, Distance, and Duration

Most experts agree EMF health risks depend on distance, duration, and distance. Refrigerators, fluorescent light fixtures, and TVs emit high levels of EMFs within twelve inches. These fall off to safe levels a few feet away. Hair dryers, shavers, and microwave ovens have high readings, but only during use. A home or school within five hundred to one thousand feet of high-tension lines or an electric power substation might have magnetic field levels between three and five mG *constantly*.

DID YOU KNOW:

- Nearly two dozen studies show electricians, power station operators, telephone linemen, and other workers exposed to electromagnetic fields have higher rates of leukemia, lymphoma, and brain cancer.[8]
- Children living near high-current power lines are almost twice as likely to develop brain tumors as children living near low-current lines.[9]
- Children born to fathers who are electricians have nearly four times the risk of developing cancer compared to other children.[10]
- The EMFs given off by a home computer terminal can be as strong as those found in homes near high-tension wires.[11]
- Home wiring improperly grounded can set off your entire plumbing system as an EMF generator.[12]
- In Sweden, there are strict regulations to limit EMF exposure. The Swedish National Board acts "on the assumption that there is a connection between exposure to power frequency magnetic fields and cancer, in particular childhood cancer."[13] What about the United States? Well, these guys built the Volvo; we built the Pinto.

SIMPLE THINGS TO DO

- Don't stand in front of the microwave oven when it's on.
- Install a grounded computer radiation screen.
- Try these substitutions:

EMF SOURCES AND SAFER ALTERNATIVES

Appliance	Safer Alternative
Hair dryer	Towel dry your hair
Electric razor	Battery-powered or safety razor

Appliance	Safer Alternative
Analog (conventional clock-face) clocks	Battery-powered clocks
Digital/electric clocks	Battery-powered clocks
Conventional electric blankets	Use only to heat bed prior to sleeping; replace with low magnetic field electric blanket.
Desk lamps with transformers	Desk lamps without transformers.
Halogen floor lamps with transformers	Halogen floor lamps without transformers
Cellular Phone	Wired phone

- Check the location of the electric circuit box. Don't sleep or sit near it, even if it is on the other side of a wall.
- Don't buy a home or send your children to a school within five hundred to one thousand feet of high-tension lines or electric power substations. If you already do, contact your local electric utility. They'll come out and measure EMFs in your home or school for free.
- Avoid buying a home with radiant heat systems in the floor or ceiling. If you already own such a home, consider replacing them.
- Buy or rent a gauss meter and take measurements throughout your home. Contact a licensed professional contractor for assistance in reducing any high EMFs.

RESOURCES

EMF Testing Equipment

Befit Enterprises, Ltd.
P.O. Box 5030
Southampton NY 11969
(800)497-9516

The Allergy Asthma Shopper

P.O. Box 239
Fate TX 75132
(800)447-1100

N.E.E.D.S.

527 Charles Avenue 12-A
Syracuse NY 13209
(800)634-1380

Baubiologie Hardware

P.O. Box 3217
Prescott AZ 86302
(602)445-8225

Computer Screens

Safe Technologies

1950 N.E. 208 Terrace
Miami FL 33179
(800) 638-9121

Non Toxic Environments

9392 S. Gribble Road
Canby OR 97013
(503)266-5244

EMF Consultants

SAGE Associates, Environmental Consultants

1283 Coast Village Circle, Suite 5
Montecito CA 93108
(805)969-0557

EMF Hot Lines

United States Environmental Protection Agency EMF Hot Line
(800)363-2384
Electric Power Research Institute Hot Line
(202)872-9222

9. ARE YOU GLOWING IN THE DARK?

As many as twenty thousand lung cancer deaths per year are caused
by radon. In some cases the amount of radon families are exposed
to is equivalent to one hundred thirty-five packs of cigarettes a day.

—EPA[1]

Dressed for success, you take a glorious gander in the mirror.
You're stunned to find you're semitransparent. You look like some
special effects audition for a Dracula movie, or Patrick Swayze in
Ghost—without Demi Moore at your side. What's going on?

It's not the ghost of Elvis. It's not some new dimension of cy-
berspace. You can't see it, touch it, taste it, smell it, but it's there,
and it can kill you. Radon is a naturally occurring radioactive gas
that breaks down into solid, radioactive particles that become
lodged in the lungs, radiating your tissues like miniature nuclear
plants. As with many other toxins, radon's health hazard builds
up over time. Certain soil and rock formations give off more radon
than others. Radon seeps out of the ground and can be sucked
into your home the way smoke is drawn up a chimney. It works
its way through cracks and joints in the foundation, and through
water drains and sump openings. Well water can bring radon right
to your kitchen or bathroom—not exactly what you expect when
you jump into your morning shower or turn on the tap to brew
your first cup of java. If your house is not well ventilated, radon
can build up in higher and higher concentrations.

Add to radon exposure the small amount of radiation given off
by your computer terminal, your TV, and those quiet radiation-
emitting smoke detectors you picked up at the local hardware
store, throw in some dental X-rays and mammograms for good
measure, and you have entered the Nuclear Age for real.

Did You Know:

- A 1988 federal survey of eleven thousand homes in seven states found one in three homes exceeded the EPA's recommended maximums for radon.[2]
- In 1990, radon was found three times more dangerous than it was estimated to be just a decade before.[3,4,5,6]
- Approximately five to ten percent of all lung cancers are related to radon exposure.[7,8]
- Radon exposure, combined with smoking, raises your risk of lung cancer fifteen times or more.[9]
- Most radon problems found in homes are easily correctable.

Simple Things to Do

- Keep your home well ventilated.
- Buy a radon detector at your local hardware store.
- If readings exceed EPA recommended levels, contact your local health department for a list of contractors qualified to remedy the problem. Often this is as simple as increasing ventilation— particularly in the basement and bathroom—sealing foundation cracks, and ventilating basement drains.
- Don't purchase hardware store ionizing smoke detectors. These have radioactive material inside. Purchase photoelectric or optical smoke detectors that have no radioactive material.
- When a dentist or doctor wants to X-ray, always question if it is actually needed. If you have doubts, get a second opinion. While it may make money for the dentist or doctor, you don't necessarily need your whole mouth X-rayed every year, or each time you change dentists. There is no proven benefit for screening premenopausal women with mammography.
- Remember, radiation builds up in the body. Reduce your exposures. Reduce your risks.

RESOURCES

Environmental Protection Agency
401 M Street S.W.
Washington, D.C. 20460
(800) 438-4318

Offers several free booklets regarding radon in homes.

Nontoxic Smoke Detectors

Baubiologie Hardware
P.O. Box 3217
Prescott AZ 86302
(602)445-8225

Ozark Water Service and Environmental Services
114 Spring St.
Sulphur Springs AR 72768
(800)835-8908

Radon Detectors

The Allergy Asthma Shopper
P.O. Box 239
Fate TX 75132
(800)447-1100

10. FREEZE 'EM, ZAP 'EM

If you want to buy any of the blood pressure or heart medications, a common antibiotic, or codeine you must see a doctor trained to write a prescription. For pesticide applicators, when you ask them

to come out to your home and spray their chemicals, the training
is minimal, toxic effects beyond the drastic are seldom mentioned,
cancer and chronic effects are not covered at all. The guy doing the
work could be illiterate.

—Janette Sherman, M.D.[1]

They'll tell you it's "safe." That it's all "EPA-approved."

We're talking about termite exterminators.

Most people think the only way to get rid of termites is to tent
and gas their homes while they hang out at the Holiday Inn for a
few days. That's like letting Saddam Hussein loose in the kid's
playroom with a fifty-five-gallon chemical drum.

Did You Know:

- For many years, the pesticide of choice for killing termites was
  chlordane. In the early 1980s, consumers looking for a termite
  treatment were assured that chlordane has an "unmatched safety
  and performance record," that it was "the safest to use." Sounds
  great! A lot of folks bought these claims hook, line, and sinker.[2]
  Today, we have some forty million homes that were sprayed with
  this stuff formerly alleged to have about as much toxicity as a
  box of crayons!
- Who paid for chlordane's propaganda blitz? Velsicol, the company manufacturing it. They're also party to chlordane-related
  lawsuits and have been banned from selling it in the United
  States.[3]
- In fact, as early as the 1940s, it was known that exposure to
  chlordane entailed "significant health hazards."[4] The killing
  power of chlordane persists for thirty years,[5] which is why it has
  been found stored in the fatty tissues of so many Americans'
  bodies. The stuff is still in all those houses.
- Chlordane is associated with cancer.[6,7,8,9] Other effects include
  blood disease, liver damage, gland dysfunction, lower immunity

to disease, birth defects, and reproductive, bone marrow, and nerve damage.[10] Yipes.

- Once chlordane was banned in 1988, exterminators turned to methyl bromide. It was said to be "safe" too. Yet studies provide evidence it causes cancer.[11,12,13] Other toxic effects include nerve, liver, kidney, and brain damage.[14] It is absorbed through the skin.

- Professional exterminators also use Vikane (sulfuryl fluoride) and chloropicrin. You don't want residues of these guys in your home, either. Vikane causes liver and kidney damage.[15] Chloropicrin causes anemia, irregular heartbeat, and asthma.[16]

- Currently, the pesticide Dursban is promoted by its manufacturer Dow Chemical Co. as a substitute for chlordane—even though the EPA has determined there are significant defects in the company's safety data.[17]

- What is known about Dursban is hardly reassuring. It is toxic to the fetus, causes nerve damage, and has been incriminated as a cause of sterility and impotency in bulls.[18] No bull.

- The EPA has requested Dow to provide additional safety information on Dursban.[19] Dow has provided zip. In fact, Dow refuses to publish its safety data for public review.[20]

- A recent study of Dursban-treated homes found the highest concentrations lower to the ground, where babies sleep and crawl.[21]

A Dubious Method for Eliminating Termites

A firefighter and his wife bought an older house they treated for termites with chlordane. He began to have headaches that lasted up to three hours and woke him up at night. In winter, his headaches became worse when the house was closed up. His wife also developed headaches. He was a hunter, storing his hunting clothes in the basement where the chlordane was applied. On a number of occasions when he was hunting, his headaches were so severe that he couldn't drive, and he had to pull off the road.

Eventually, he suffered a blackout spell and was hospitalized. After an investigation, his home was found to be so contaminated with chlordane, it had to be demolished. That's not the way you want to get rid of termites.[22]

Simple Things to Do

The use of alternative termite controls can be as cost-effective as pesticides for elimination of dry-wood termites.

- Professional contractors can simply raise the heat in a home to about one hundred twenty degrees. This will kill ninety-nine percent of the buggers. Fry, baby, fry.
- Liquid nitrogen sprayed into the wall will freeze termites' tiny buns off and eliminate virtually all of them.
- Microwave techniques can zap about ninety-two percent.
- Electric shock, administered by electro-guns, nails about eighty percent of the little criminals. Now that's capital punishment.

  Prevention is important:

- Make sure that none of the wood parts of your home come into contact with the soil.
- When building a house, remodeling, or renovating, use select-harvested redwood, cedar, cypress, oak, or Douglas fir. All have some resistance to termites.[23,24]
- Coarse sand, around the foundation or in crawl spaces, makes an effective barrier. Termites can't walk through it.[25]
- Remove food sources such as tree stumps, construction debris, and buried wood from underneath the home or near the foundation—no more free lunch.
- Minimize the moisture in the wood, particularly wood close to the ground.
- Outside the home, have downspouts take water several feet away from the house.
- For treatment of subterranean termites, try nematodes (particularly *Steinernema feltiae, Neoaplacenta carpocapsae,* and *Hetero-habditis heliothis*) to control them.[26] Studies show these warriors

kill ninety-six percent of damp-wood termites and ninety-eight percent of wood-dwelling termites within three days.[27]

RESOURCES

Bio-Integral Resource Center

P.O. Box 7414
Berkeley CA 94707
(415)524-2567

A nonprofit corporation undertaking research and education in integrated pest management and least toxic pest control. Many booklets available for nominal fees.

Ecola Services Inc.

(800)332-BUGS

Electro-gun termite control.

The Green Spot, Ltd.

Department of Bio-Ingenuity
93 Priest Road
Barrington NH 03825-6204
(603)942-8925
Fax: (603)942-8932

Excellent selection of a wide range of nematodes for termite control as well as practical advice. Their Green Methods™ catalog is an excellent resource publication and worth having. It is free.

Tallon

1949 East Market St.
Long Beach CA 90805
(800)779-2653

Nitrogen termite control. Other least toxic controls.

11. I PROMISE YOU A ROSE GARDEN

It's easy to grow gardens once you learn a few tricks of the nontoxic trade. And what you get along the way is a much greater opportunity for you and your family to stay healthy. Live a few more years. Avoid cancer. Things like that.

Many of the pesticides sold in garden shops are indiscriminate "shotgun killers." They wipe out both plant pests—which make up only a small proportion of the total insects in your garden—*and* ninety percent of the rest of the insects, which are largely beneficial and help to control pests.[1] They also might wipe out you.

DID YOU KNOW:

- One study found a rate of childhood leukemia four to seven times greater in children whose parents used store-bought home and garden pesticides.[2]
- Childhood brain cancer is tied to use of Diazinon, carbaryl (Sevin), and weed killers.[3]
- There is a relationship between insecticides and weed killers and leukemia.[4]
- Of the thirty-four most commonly used lawn chemicals, eleven are known to cause cancer; twenty, nervous system poisoning; nine, birth defects; and thirty, skin irritation.[5]

SIMPLE THINGS TO DO

- Say good-bye to toxic pesticides; say hello to *Bacillus thuringiensis (Bt)*, fatty acid soaps, sulfur, and superior horticultural oils, and, of course, a host of "good" bugs. Here are some of the best least toxic methods to control garden pests.

NATURAL GARDENING ALTERNATIVES TO TOXIC PESTICIDES

Alternative	*Diseases/Pests Attacked*	*Comments*
Microorganisms		
Bacillus thuringiensis (Bt)	Beetles, caterpillars, fungus gnats, and mosquitoes.	Use as dust, liquid, powder, or granules.
Nosema locustae	Crickets and grasshoppers.	Long-term control.[6]
Nematodes		
Heterorhabditis bacteriophora	Billbugs, black vine weevils, corn rootworm larvae, Japanese beetle grubs, masked chafers, mole crickets, and wireworms.	Repeated releases work best.[7]
Steinernema carpocapsae	Carpenterworms, cutworms, currant borers, earwigs, fungus gnats, navel orangeworms, onion maggots, pillbugs, seedcorn maggots, sod webworms, sowbugs, and strawberry root weevils.	See above.
Insects		
Aphid midge (*Aphidoletes aphidimyza*)[8]	Aphids (more than 60 species, excluding melon aphids).[9]	Release at rate of about 1 cocoon per square foot.
Lacewing (various species)[10]	Aphids especially, possible predator of caterpillars, mealybugs, mites, moth eggs, scales, thrips.[11]	Generally release 5 per square foot weekly or biweekly.

Alternative	Diseases/Pests Attacked	Comments
Insects		
Ladybugs (*Hippodamia convergens*)	Aphids.	Release in evening after watering foliage at the rate of 1–2 beetles per square foot. Small repeated releases work best.
Trichogramma wasps (various species)[12]	More than 200 species of moths.	Generally used at rate of 5,000 to 7,000 per infested tree, applied every 5 to 7 days during moth flying season.
Whitefly parasite (*Encarsia formosa*)[13]	Greenhouse whiteflies.[14]	Release 1 per square foot weekly or biweekly. Repeat releases a must.
Chemical Controls		
Diatomaceous earth[15]	Soft-bodied pests such as ants and aphids.[16]	Dust over, around plants.[17] Wear dust mask to avoid inhaling powder.
Fatty acid herbicidal and insecticidal soaps	Aphids, chinch bugs, crab grass, dandelions, flea beetles, mealybugs, sod webworms, thrips, whiteflies. Also small weeds.	Spray soapy liquid on infested plants, weeds.

Alternative Chemical Control	Diseases/Pests Attacked	Comments
Sulfur[18]	Black spot, brown rot, fungus, mites, powdery mildew, rust.[19]	Can be dusted or mixed with water and sprayed. Wear dust mask and protective gloves when applying. Never dust against wind.[20]
Physical Controls		
Slug and snail traps	Slugs and snails.	Generally, 1 trap per 10 square feet. Best when partially buried in soil.

• Select a supplier who will take the time to discuss your individual pest control needs.

RESOURCES

The Green Spot, Ltd.
Department of Bio-Ingenuity
93 Priest Road
Barrington NH 03825-6204
(603)942-8925
Fax: (603)942-8932

Excellent selection of a wide range of natural pest controls in all categories. Their Green Methods™ catalog is an excellent resource publication and worth having.

Canada
Applied Bio-Nomics, Ltd.
11074 West Saanich Road
Sydney, British Columbia, Canada V8L 5P5
(604)656-2123

Excellent selection of biological pest control agents.

12. MY LIFE AS A DOG

"Tick and flea dips . . . contain a variety of active ingredients and solvents that might cause cancer in animals. Furthermore, each time a pet animal is treated with a tick and flea dip, substantial human exposure is likely to occur, primarily by absorption through the skin while handling the pet."

—NATIONAL RESEARCH COUNCIL[1]

It's not the sleeping on the floor that bothers me, or drinking out of that disgusting toilet. I don't even mind the little brats pulling my ears. I can play dumb and feed my condescending master's ego—even though my IQ is fifteen points higher. (He's an OK guy.) I can even pretend to like the table scraps—even if no self-respecting canine would admit eating half-eaten succotash and mashed potatoes. But the one thing I can't stand, the one thing that has to stop, is being sprayed and dunked with that flea stuff. Heck, that bitch, Susie, next door has been in heat all week and I can't perform.

Psst, psst: Hey, Fido. If it is any consolation, the guy dousing you with all those chemicals can't perform either and he doesn't have a clue what the real problem is.

Many of us have grown up thinking all we need to do is run down to the corner supermarket, purchase flea spray, and "bomb" our pets and home—the old "nuke 'em" theory.[2] In fact, when it comes to controlling fleas and ticks, you may love your pet and want to help, but you could end up loving your pet to death. It's time to stop poisoning Felix, Fido, Frank, Franny, and the rest of the freaking family!

DID YOU KNOW:

- RED ALERT: Some pesticides commonly used in flea and tick products cause cancer.[3,4,5,6,7,8]
- The pesticide carbaryl, commonly used in pet flea and tick killers, causes birth defects in dogs.[9]
- Cats constantly lick their fur and, if treated with chemicals, can consume a lot more poison than dogs.[10]
- The EPA reports that Hartz Mountain Blockade, containing two powerful pesticides, is responsible for over two hundred known dog and cat poisonings. The label for Blockade warns pets may experience salivation, tremors, or vomiting upon application.[11]
- Bladder cancer in dogs is associated with lifetime exposure to tick and flea dips.[12]
- Childhood brain cancer is associated with flea collars on pets and home pesticide "bombs."[13]
- People applying flea and tick dips can suffer muscle weakness and tingling of the extremities.[14] People who "dust" pets with powders are likely to suffer nausea and headaches. People who chemically sponge pets may suffer convulsions and mental confusion.[15]
- Flea foggers and bombs expose everyone and everything in the house to toxic chemicals. Some are flammable, making their use around appliances with pilot lights dangerous.[16] (Don't blow yourself up; we like you.)
- Limonene (also known as d-limonene) in flea sprays can cause vomiting, nausea, salivation, muscle tremors, staggering, imbalance, and other symptoms of nervous system poisoning. It is especially hazardous when used on cats,[17] but should not be used on dogs either. Moreover, limonene is suspected of causing cancer, birth defects, kidney damage, and harm to the immune system.[18]

SIMPLE THINGS TO DO

- Shampoos are safest. Flea shampoos are *not* associated with skin irritation or nerve poisoning.[19] We particularly recommend fatty acid soaps, purchased from pet shops or garden nurseries. When shampooing, leave the soap in your pet's coat for a half hour and then rinse. It suffocates the fleas.[20]

- Use a flea comb, available at pet stores. Drown them in soapy water.
- One way to avoid flea bombs is to use an outside flea service, such as FleaBusters, that uses safe materials.[21]
- Try vacuuming. It's simple and helps eliminate eggs. Immediately remove and seal the bag.[22]
- Don't use flea sprays that contain limonene.
- Safer products contain methoprene (Precor) and hydroprene that stop eggs from hatching. The best time to use these is before flea season, in the spring. Fleas lay eggs when the temperature is over sixty-five degrees.[23]
- For lawn fleas, a nontoxic alternative is to use nematodes. These tiny worms can be sprayed on lawns and they will kill flea larvae.
- Fleas are attracted to dry, chapped skin. Primrose oil mixed with pet food has been shown to help heal rashes.[24] Aloe vera leaf, rubbed on inflamed areas, also helps.

Nutritional Flea Control

Although some hopeful pet owners believe feeding their pets yeast will repel fleas, experts report little to no success.[25] On the other hand, there is some evidence that feeding pets garlic helps.[26] Feed pets one clove of crushed raw garlic daily for each ten pounds of body weight or use garlic extract available at drug stores. When using a garlic extract, feed two capsules for each ten pounds of body weight.[27] Hey, his breath might not be great, but you'll get rid of those little vampires!

RESOURCES

Biosys
1057 E. Meadow Circle
Palo Alto CA 94303
(415)856-9500

Nematodes.

Farnam Pet Products
P.O. Box 34820
Phoenix AZ 85067

Nematodes; free flea control video.

FleaBusters
655 N.W. 9th Avenue
Suite 412
Fort Lauderdale FL 33309
(800)765-FLEA

Nontoxic in-home flea eradication.

The Natural Pet Care Company
2713 East Madison
Seattle WA 98112
(800)962-8266

Least toxic flea control products.

Wow-Bow Distributors
13B Lucon Drive
Deer Park NY 11729
(516)254-6064
(800)326-0230

Least toxic flea control products.

13. ATTACK OF THE KILLER HOUSE . . .

BUILDING IT BETTER

A five-year study by the United States Environmental Protection Agency found levels of toxic pollutants one hundred to two hundred times higher indoors than outdoors.[1]

John Belushi isn't lurking in a corner opening beer bottles with his teeth; there's no food fight in the kitchen, and there are no fraternity coeds squirming and wiggling on the den floor. No, you don't live in *Animal House*. But that den of iniquity and your home have one thing in common—they can both make you sick!

Take a building. Fill it with synthetic chemicals, radioactive gases, chemically treated wood, dust, bacteria, cans of pesticides and other toxins, and even some devices giving off radiation. Insulate it. Paint it. For good measure, put a tent over it and gas it. You have just built the good old American home—heck, it looks like an Exxon oil spill! Maybe that's why an EPA scientist says only half-jokingly, "Even downwind from a chemical plant, it's better to open your windows."[2]

DID YOU KNOW:

- The National Research Council reports that fifteen percent of the United States population has an increased sensitivity to chemicals commonly found in the home.[3]
- About 40 pounds of dust settles in the average United States home each year.[4] And we thought Charlie Brown had it bad with Pigpen!
- Gas and oil heaters, gas ranges and dryers, kerosene heaters, and wood stoves give off carbon monoxide, carbon dioxide, sulfur

dioxide, and nitrogen dioxide. Symptoms of poisoning include impaired vision and thinking, nausea, loss of judgment, dizziness, headaches, and weakness. Anyone have a gas mask?

- A gas oven operating at three hundred and fifty degrees for one hour with an exhaust fan can cause indoor air pollution comparable to a heavy Los Angeles smog.[5]
- People drinking hard water, rather than soft, have less likelihood of a heart attack.[6,7] Hard water provides higher levels of calcium and magnesium, which are generally good for your heart. Softened water can have high levels of sodium chloride (salt), which can be harmful to your heart.
- Up to eight percent of the population is sensitive to formaldehyde. Six billion pounds of formaldehyde are produced annually,[8,9] much of it for home use.[10,11]
- An attached or garage under the house can release petroleum fumes into the home. Fumes can cause headaches, allergies, and fatigue.
- Formaldehyde is found in particleboard furniture and cabinets, plywood, fiberglass, fiberboard, and paneling.[12]
- Old, popcorn ceiling plaster or white insulation pipe covers often contain asbestos, which causes lung cancer. It kills nine to twelve thousand Americans every year.[13]
- Homes with southern and eastern light exposure are cooler in summer. The sunlight kills mold and mildew for free.

SIMPLE THINGS TO DO

- Use wood rather than plastic blinds, which give off fumes when hot.
- Leave the garage door open as much as possible, if you have an attached or underneath garage. If air ducts connect to the home, seal them off.
- Have your water tested. If toxins are found, or if the water is chlorinated, filter the drinking water (see Chapter 27).
- Disconnect the water softener.
- Replace gas appliances with electric ones. Start with the oven and stove.
- Seal or replace particleboard walls, floors or cabinets.

- Store household chemicals outside in a ventilated garage or storage shed.
- Clean the area near your furnace. Make sure there is a fresh air supply coming in and exhaust air is vented out. Inspect and seal fuel leaks.
- Increase southern and eastern morning light into your home.

RESOURCES

Nontoxic Building Materials

Thoroseal
Standard Dry Wall Products
7800 N.W. 38th Street
Miami FL 33166

Particleboard sealer
Crystal Aire I
Pace Industries, Inc.
779 S. La Grange Avenue
Newbury Park CA 91320
(805)499-2911

Heating & cooling systems
Thurmond Development Corp.
P.O. Box 23037
Little Rock AR 72211
(800)AIR-PURE

Insulation
Air-Krete Inc.
P.O. Box 380
Weedsport NY 13166
(315)834-6609

Certainteed Corporation
P.O. Box 860
Valley Forge PA 19482
(215)341-7000

Asbestos Information

Asbestos Information Center
Tufts University, Curtis Hall
Medford MA 02155
(617)381-3486

Consumer Product Safety Commission
1111 18th St. N.W.
Washington DC 20207
(800)638-2772

14. THE AMERICAN DREAM

No house is perfect. But the place with the most checks is where you want to be.

- ☐ No high-tension power lines, TV transmitters, or microwave relay stations within one-half mile (see Chapter 8).
- ☐ No asbestos ceilings or pipes.
- ☐ No blocked eastern sunlight.
- ☐ No plastic or galvanized plumbing—copper preferred.
- ☐ No urea-formaldehyde foam, fiberglass, or cellulose insulation.
- ☐ No lead-based paint, inside or out.
- ☐ No toxic waste operations in area over the last fifty years (check with local health department and EPA records of designed hazardous waste sites).
- ☐ No basement.
- ☐ No chlordane or other chemical termite treatments in the past ten to twenty years.
- ☐ No carpeting over particleboard floors—hardwood or tile preferred.
- ☐ No particleboard or pressed-wood cabinets—hardwood or metal preferred.

☐ No attached or underneath garage.

☐ No basement oil or gas heaters (prefer these located outside the house).

☐ No gas ovens, ranges, dryers, or hot water heaters.

☐ No foundation cracks.

☐ No farms (spraying pesticides) or freeways nearby.

☐ No medium to high radon levels (see Chapter 9).

☐ No valley location in a congested area.

☐ No toxic metals, chlorinated solvents, or other contaminants in a complete water analysis (see Chapter 27).

☐ No water softener.

☐ No gas or oil furnace in basement—an electric forced air heating/cooling system with heat exchange ventilator preferred.

☐ No high EMF readings inside or outside (see Chapter 8).

☐ No newly tarred roof near open windows.

☐ No new oil-based paints on interior walls.

Happy Hunting!!

15. HONEY, THERE'S A MONSTER IN THE POOL!

Pour in muriatic acid, dump in polyoxyethylene, sprinkle some chlorine and cyanuric acid for seasoning, top off with soda ash, and stir well. No, you're not mixing the latest summer fad cocktail or concocting a voodoo brew to cast a spell on the postman for being late with your mail for the last five days. You're dumping in your pool what most of us do. Then you're going to jump and swim in, and swallow, this brew.

DID YOU KNOW:

• Cyanuric acid, linked to kidney and bladder problems, is used as a chlorine stabilizer in most swimming pools. An EPA risk assessment suggests swimmers are at risk from levels commonly found in pools.[1]

- A study found ninety-two percent of competitive swimmers had breathing problems caused by chemicals in the pool.[2]
- Chlorine and cyanuric acid are absorbed through the skin as you swim. They are also inhaled.[3]
- Chlorine combines with organic material in a pool to form a family of cancer-causing chemicals, trihalomethanes.
- The high heat of hot tubs can cause birth defects, particularly during early pregnancy.[4]

SIMPLE THINGS TO DO

- Install a pool ozonator or ultraviolet light system to kill bacteria. An extra benefit of this method is your eyes won't get bloodshot.
- Regularly maintain and run your filter system to help reduce your need for chlorine and other chemicals.
- Ask your local public pool to investigate nontoxic effective alternatives to dousing the water with toxic chemicals.

RESOURCES

Pool Ozone and Ultraviolet Light Systems

DEL Industries
3428 Bullock Lane
San Luis Obispo CA 93401
(800)676-1335

Least Toxic Pool Supplies

Natural Chemistry, Inc.
244 Elm St.
New Canaan CT 06840
(800)753-1233

Part II

THE WHOLE FAMILY FEELING GOOD

---

16. JUST SAY NO!

"Marijuana depresses every function in the body—energy level, thinking, sperm count, testosterone, ovulation—and since the body can't get rid of marijuana's chief chemicals . . . the damage goes on and on."

—ROY HART, M.D.[1]

We wanted to think of something funny to tell you about drugs. There isn't. The tragic and devastating consequences of drug abuse have been thoroughly documented. However, you probably don't know many drugs, legal and illegal, are stored in your body LONG after you cease using them.[2,3,4,5,6] Stored drug residues can adversely affect your health.

DID YOU KNOW:

- THC, the active ingredient in marijuana, stays in the body longer than the pesticide DDT. The marijuana smoked in the 1960s was one-half percent THC. Today, competing with other street drugs, marijuana is ten to fourteen percent THC. Studies show that marijuana damages the lungs more than tobacco and contains cancer-causing chemicals.[7] Marijuana causes brain damage.[8,9] One marijuana joint a day damages the lungs as much as smoking a pack of cigarettes a day.[10,11]

- LSD and various "designer drugs" reduce oxygen to the brain and damage it.[12]
- Angel dust, cocaine, LSD, Valium, and even alcohol have all been shown in scientific studies to store in the body's tissue after use.[13,14,15,16,17,18,19,20,21]
- Drugs stored in the fat tissues move into the bloodstream during periods of stress, exercise, or dieting.[22]
- This combination of buildup in the tissues and movement into the bloodstream explains in part the phenomena of "flashbacks" where a person off drugs, for months or even years, reexperiences a drug "trip," frequently never quite feeling right.[23] This can also cause cravings and is associated with the high rate of people going back on drugs after successfully coming off them. The drugs are still in their system!
- There are up to forty thousand hospital admissions every year from bad drug reactions.

COMPARATIVE CAUSES OF DEATH: ANNUAL AVERAGES IN UNITED STATES[24,25]	
Adverse drug reactions	60,000–140,000
Heart attacks	75,000
Automobile accidents	39,325
Hair dryer accidents	10
Vitamin overdoses	0

- Legally prescribed drugs can also be hazardous to your health. A drug investigator evaluating drug safety for a pharmaceutical company can be paid one thousand dollars per patient studied and make upwards of one million dollars a year. How much repeat business is there if he finds a drug to be unsafe?[26,27]
- Drug reactions account for as many as fifty million hospital days per year.[28]

- Many commonly prescribed drugs cause or promote cancer. These include high blood pressure medications, antibiotics, and tranquilizers. The antidepressants Elavil and Prozac increase tumor growth rate in rodents.[29]

Some That Definitely Won't Turn You On . . .

Drugs can adversely affect your sexual function. Chief among these are antidepressants such as Prozac, Nardil, Desyrel, Parnate, and some blood pressure medications.[30]

Take a Number

Adverse drug reactions reported to the FDA.[31,32]

Drug	Number Reported	Years Reported
Elavil	2,923	21 years
Valium	6,343	21 years
Prozac	14,184	3 years

SIMPLE THINGS TO DO

- Don't use illegal drugs. They'll kill you fast or slow. For real!
- Don't take prescribed or over-the-counter drugs without your doctor's recommendation or consulting a recent edition of the *Physicians' Desk Reference*.
- Take no drugs—street, prescribed, or over-the-counter—if you are pregnant without first consulting your physician.
- Find a doctor knowledgeable in nutritional AND traditional medicine. Examine safer alternatives to drugs with your doctor. Use proven, safe nutritional and homeopathic remedies.
- Do a detoxification program to flush out drug residues if you have a history of illegal or prescription drug abuse. Remember, drug residues store in the body and can affect you later (see Chapter 20).

• .Women who used drugs can go through a detoxification program before pregnancy.

RESOURCES

American College for Advancement in Medicine

23121 Verdugo Drive, Suite 204
Laguna Hills CA 92653
(800)532-3688
(714)583-7666
(714)455-9679 Fax

A nutritionally oriented college of physicians with members across the United States and Canada. Provides physician names in your area.

Narconon International

6381 Hollywood Blvd.
Los Angeles CA 90010
(213)962-2404

Provides international education and rehabilitation services, including resident drug rehabilitation programs and detoxification.

17. WHAT'S UP, DOC?

"There is widespread agreement that with few exceptions physicians are inadequately trained in occupational and environmental medicine."

—NATIONAL ACADEMY OF SCIENCES[1]

Fred's had lingering headaches for five years. His family doctor said it's due to stress but gave Fred a $1000 brain scan anyway—"just to be sure." It showed zilch. Fred refused the prescription for the painkillers and figured the psychiatrist his doctor recommended would only add to his stress. There is enough stress in Fred's life. His office, for example. The building is awfully stuffy, and ever since the boss let his wife move in her cosmetics business it smells funny. But Fred doesn't say anything—as long as they keep giving him that indoor parking spot. Heck, by the end of the day, Fred almost feels high. Fred's biggest stress at home is not having his own space for his favorite hobby, oil painting life-size plaster busts of Richard Nixon. He has to share the garage with his wife, who refinishes furniture she collects from the Salvation Army dumpster. The stuff she uses smells pretty bad but Fred has to keep the doors and windows closed to keep out the dust. Fred's biggest recent financial stress is the exterminator's bill. He got a free termite inspection and they discovered the house was infested and had to be sprayed for a week. Fred's headaches were getting worse. An office temp sporting purple, spiked hair and four-inch black porcelain nails told Fred about a doctor turned psychic-healer. Fred decided he had nothing to lose and gave the guy a try. The "healer's" office looked like a cross between the set for *Little Shop of Horrors* and an herb garden rummage sale. The guy looked a little like Rodney Dangerfield, which didn't bother Fred half as much as his nose ring and the Ouija board on his desk. Sadly, this Rodney Dangerfield lookalike might have better luck than Fred's own doctor figuring out that chemicals are causing Fred's problems.

If you or a family member were suffering from symptoms of a low-level toxic exposure, your family doctor might not have a clue of the potential causes for your problems. Family doctors receive little training in environmental medicine. Although your doctor knows what to do if your child drinks something from under the kitchen sink, most doctors know almost nothing about health effects from low-level exposure that can come from toxins in drinking water, household products, or smog. They know even less about prevention and treating these kinds of conditions.[2]

This puts you at risk. Headaches, blurred vision, allergies, asthma, skin irritations, hyperactivity, tremors, fatigue, numbness in your fingers and toes, lowered IQ, inability to concentrate, memory loss, depression, and irritability are all symptoms caused by low-level toxic exposure and often misdiagnosed by doctors.

Doctors, expected to have the answer, often label a complaint "psychological" when they don't know what the real answer is and refer you to a psychologist or a psychiatrist. This can worsen your condition not only because you are not getting the proper treatment to the underlying cause, but because you have an undiagnosed chemical exposure and you may be prescribed more chemicals.

DID YOU KNOW:

- Fewer than two thousand of the half-million physicians in the United States are certified in occupational medicine.[3]
- Many Americans have high enough lead levels in their bodies to cause lowered IQ, hyperactivity, high blood pressure, skin and stomach problems, and reproductive damage. Few are screened for this hazard.
- Symptoms from DDT, chlordane, dieldrin, and PCBs can be treated, but necessary blood tests to detect these chemicals are rarely done.

SIMPLE THINGS TO DO

- Ask your doctor to do a "solvent screen" blood test if you work with toxic chemicals or use them frequently around your home.
- Ask your doctor to run a "pesticide screen" blood test if you have lived on a farm, worked with agricultural chemicals, had your house treated for termites, or use home and garden pesticides—and you're feeling sick. There are two major groups of pesticides: organophosphates and organochlorines.
- Have your breast milk tested if you are planning to have children and breast-feed them and have worked with, or lived around, pesticides. While the benefits from breast-feeding almost always outweigh the risks, some women could have dangerously high levels of contaminants in their breast milk.[4,5] These levels can be reduced (see Chapter 20).

- Discuss with your doctor tests that measure IQ, memory, and reaction time to detect problems caused by chemicals, if you have reason to be concerned about a toxic exposure.
- Discuss with your doctor blood tests that measure the immune system and its reaction to common toxic chemicals, if you are concerned about your immunity after a chemical exposure.

RESOURCES

The American Academy of Environmental Medicine

4510 West 89th Street
Prairie Village KS 66207
(913)642-6062

A medical academy that can refer physicians in your area who diagnose and treat chemical exposures and sensitivities in patients.

Laboratories for Analyzing Body Burdens of Toxins

Accu-Chem Laboratory

990 N. Bowser Road, Suite 800
Richardson TX 75081
(800)451-0116

Performs solvent, pesticide, and heavy metal screens on blood and urine.

National Medical Services

2300 Stratford Avenue
Willow Grove PA 19090
(215)657-4900

Performs solvent, pesticide, and heavy metal screens on blood and urine.

Pacific Toxicology Laboratory

1541 Pontius Avenue
Los Angeles CA 90025
(310)479-4911

Performs solvent, pesticide, and heavy metal screens on blood and urine.

Other Tests

Antibody Assay Lab

1715 East Wilshire, Suite 715
Santa Ana CA 92705
(714)972-9979

Performs immune system tests to measure chemical exposures.

Kaye Kilburn, M.D.

University of Southern California Medical School
2250 Alcazar St., Room 201
Los Angeles CA 90033
(213)342-1830

Performs tests for balance, blink reflex, reaction time, memory, and IQ after a chemical exposure.

Neuro-Test, Inc.

3250 Mesaloa Lane
Pasadena, CA 91107
(no phone)

Performs tests for balance, blink reflex, reaction time, memory, and IQ after a chemical exposure.

18. A Phytomin a Day Keeps

the Toxins Away

"Supplementation and fortification of the diet with antioxidant vitamins and minerals could become an effective strategy for cancer control."

—Tim Byers and Geraldine Perry[1]

At thirty-six, Scott Miller's largest health concern is preventing cancer. His father and grandfather died of cancer; so did his brother. Indeed, it is Miller's fear of the big "C" and his need to feel he is doing *something* that led him several years ago to begin a program of daily supplements. Although his intention is good, are vitamins, supplements, and herbal remedies the only solution? Are we supposed to stuff fifty-eight vitamin pills down our throat every day and chase them with some exotic tea made from the sweat and urine of a Tibetan llama? Not likely.

Everyone is concerned about cancer. There are numerous reports and claims that appear in magazines and on TV and radio about vitamins, herbs, and other substances that can either prevent or cure cancer. These claims are sometimes overly exuberant and reflect the pitfalls of both capitalism and the free market. While some claims may be unsubstantiated, there are in fact vitamins, minerals, and other substances that may help prevent cancer. One aspect of cancer prevention is called "chemoprevention." One of the most exciting new developments in nutrition is the identification of the "phytomin." While the health benefits from vitamin and mineral supplementation have been known for years, scientists have long believed that the disease-preventing properties in certain foods are not just single vitamins or minerals. Healthy vegetables, fruits, and other plants contain thousands of potential disease-preventing substances. Nutritional supplements have been developed from whole plant foods, thus retaining a wider range of their potentially beneficial properties. These are called "phytomins." Additional research is needed to understand their full benefits but "phytomins" are available.

DID YOU KNOW:

- Evidence that dietary supplements help prevent cancer is accumulating. There have been only some thirty-five randomized large-scale studies, testing a wide range of substances. Results from twenty-eight of these were reported only in the last five years, but have raised tremendous interest in the use of supplements for cancer prevention.[2,3]

- Early use of supplements *before* cancer is crucial for their optimal effectiveness.
- Exposure to low levels of environmental toxins ("free radicals") that damage DNA (the body's "blueprint" for orderly cell growth) "might well be the underlying cause of . . . increased incidence of cancer and other diseases of old age."[4] Supplements help prevent cancer by protecting DNA.
- A poor diet may decrease the body's own ability to eliminate certain toxins.[5] Many people suffer deficiencies of nutrients such as vitamins B_6, B_{12}, C, D, and E, all known to help rid the body of toxins.[6]
- Beta-carotene is thought to prevent lung cancer in humans by preventing DNA damage. Hundreds of others of its chemical cousins are found in fruits and vegetables and may be the real heroes when it comes to disease prevention.
- Data suggests that supplementing your diet with vitamin C may also protect against the body's accumulation of cancer-causing metals such as cadmium.[7] As with beta-carotene, vitamin C is found packed in foods along with closely related chemical "cousins," bioflavonoids. Vitamin C and bioflavonoids may well work better together than alone.
- Garlic pills are another part of many cancer-prevention programs, especially among women. In an animal study, investigators reported that both regular garlic and garlic enriched with selenium (a trace mineral) significantly inhibited breast cancers.[8,9]

What's All This Fuss About Melatonin?

Melatonin is the name of a hormone (a substance produced in the body by a gland) secreted by the pineal gland near the brain. Darkness and the body's daily time clock trigger its nightly secretions. Levels of melatonin decline with aging. Keeping up levels of the hormone as people age is thought by some to help prevent a wide range of diseases and conditions from cancer to sleeplessness. Melatonin may have the power to alter the body's time clock. In scientific experiments in Switzerland, old rats receiving this hormone stayed younger, longer. It has shown potential anticancer properties in rodent studies. Melatonin has only been available recently in stores after vitamin companies learned how to make it inexpensively. Pills or drops are taken under the tongue in one- to six-milligram doses, though most recommendations advise the lower-end dose. It seems safe, although it might not be appropriate to use it every day. Its primary, and practical, use is to assist sleep in travelers who change time zones and suffer from jet lag. There are some health conditions which indicate not using melatonin. Always consult your physician before taking it or any drug. For further reading there are many popular books currently available. Its long-term effects, which appear positive at this time, are not yet definitely known.[10]

Simple Things to Do

- There is nothing that can replace an optimal diet rich in fresh fruits, vegetables, and whole grains. But if you are like President Bush and don't eat your broccoli, a vitamin a day may keep the doctor away, even though it won't get you reelected. Supplementing with a few extra pills a day, containing extracts of herbs and other plant chemicals, is a sensible and inexpensive insurance policy.
- Look into "phytomins" such as garlic, grapeseed extract, and flavonoids (found in the same fruits and vegetables as vitamin C).

The Four ACES—A Winning Hand

If you're going to supplement, it is important that you start with a basic program, consisting of the ACES, vitamins A, C, E, and selenium. Certain toxins in the body can change normally harmless molecules into irritants that can damage your cells. This harmful process is called "oxidation." The irritants that are created in this process are called "free radicals." Hence, vitamins and minerals which neutralize these irritants are called antioxidants. Generally, natural-source vitamins have greater potency. Make sure that your supplements are balanced and contain B-complex vitamins and vitamin D, as well as minerals such as calcium and magnesium. For a vitamin A source, be sure to seek natural source beta-carotene, which provides a mix of its chemical cousins, too.

Tea for Two

Studies have shown that lower incidence of certain cancers in Japan has been associated with daily use of green tea, which is rich in antioxidants.[11,12] Hold the java, have a cup of tea, and drink to your health!

19. GET SMART!

Your child's IQ has been lowered two to eight points by environmental exposure to lead.[1]

Your son forgets his lunch. He forgets his report card, which you'd like to, since it was mostly C's and D's, anyway. He forgets your name! He goes from being so hyper that you're looking for that tranquilizer dart gun they used on *Wild Kingdom* to being so lethargic he's watching slow-motion instant replays with the pause button *on*. You start examining his pupils. You have him drug tested. He's "clean." You're convinced it's all your fault as you wait for a call from the producer of *Sally Jessy Raphael* asking you to appear with your son who has written them accusing you of making him play truth or dare with you and imaginary pygmies. Before you panic, consider that he might have just hit hyperspace from exposure to environmental toxins.[2,3,4]

All the problems plaguing our young people today can't be pinned on toxic chemicals. The failure of modern education is, in no small part, linked to the introduction in the 1950s of "modern psychology" into education, an approach that fails to acknowledge the moral human spirit, reducing young people and their responsibilities to a "feel good" mentality and turning classroom education into another venue for stimulus-response control techniques. Treat a child like a rat in a cage, and that's how he'll act. It's OK to drug rats. This denial of a young person's responsibility, creativity, and ability has promoted cockeyed solutions such as "Only do it if it feels good" and "Get in touch with your feelings." It wasn't a schoolyard drug pusher who first chanted "Tune in, turn on, drop out"—but a Harvard University psychologist. Still, there is no denying the damaging role of industrial pollution and drugs on a child's ability to learn.

DID YOU KNOW:

- Behavioral problems may be the earliest sign of low-level chemical exposure. A childhood behavioral expert has observed: "Accumulating evidence has led some researchers to the hypothesis that the academic and behavioral problems seen in American youth are the result of subtle biological factors which include impairment of the brain by lead, food additives, other toxic substances, food sensitivities and improper nutrition. . . . For 9 years I was the Chairman of the Scientific Studies Committee of the Association for Children and Adults with Learning Disabilities. That experience . . . has convinced me that environmental pollution and what we eat can definitely adversely affect thinking ability."[5]
- Hyperactivity and attention deficit disorder are altogether too commonly diagnosed in kids today. Children across the country are put on the drug Ritalin to control these disorders when, unfortunately, the real culprits may be lead and other chemicals that build up in a child's body, causing learning and behavioral problems.[6] How many parents, doctors, and educators are aware of this? Instead of finding the environmental cause, the child is put on a drug, adding another chemical to the mix.
- Artificial dyes such as red dye number 3 and tartrazine, artificial

sweeteners, food preservatives, and pesticides can cause behavioral disorders.[7,8,9,10]

- Studies have shown that the nervous system and a child's IQ can improve if chemicals are eliminated from the body.[11]
- "The National Academy of Sciences recently reported that twelve percent of the sixty-three million children under the age of eighteen in the United States suffer from one or more mental disorders. The report identified exposure to toxic substances before or after birth as one of the several risk factors that appear to make children vulnerable . . ."[12]
- Less than ten percent of the seventy thousand everyday chemicals have been tested for their toxic effects on the nervous system.[13]
- Five percent of children under the age of six (one million preschoolers) have blood levels that exceed standards.[14]
- Glazed ceramics and leaded glass crystal contain lead that can leach into your children's food or drink. Some manufacturers now produce safe glassware and ceramics and will provide you with information.
- Children are more vulnerable to toxic chemicals than adults. Their brain's protective barrier is less well developed, allowing more toxins to pass through and cause damage.[15,16]
- Many chemicals found in cleaning compounds, waxes, glues, paints, and other products used in homes and schools are easily inhaled and absorbed through the skin and lungs. Their primary target is the brain.[17]

SIMPLE THINGS TO DO

- Get yourself and your kids on a healthy diet (see Chapters 22 through 32).
- Insist that your school serve safe and healthy foods. If not, have your children "brown bag it."
- Go to your child's school and find out what chemicals and products are used for painting, cleaning, construction, and pest control. Insist on safer alternatives, if necessary (see Chapters 4 through 10 and 13).

- Make sure your child's school is tested for lead (see Chapters 17 and 27).
- Do a lead test for your child (see Chapter 17).
- If your child's lead test result is high, discuss chelation or detoxification with your doctor (see Chapter 20).
- Don't store liquids in leaded glass crystal.
- Have a change room where work clothes are discarded before going into the home if you or your spouse works with chemicals on the job.
- Avoid household pesticides. Use safer alternatives (see Chapters 10 through 13).

RESOURCES

Alliance to End Childhood Lead Poisoning

600 Pennsylvania Ave. S.E., Suite 100
Washington DC 20003
(202)543-1147

Public education, technical assistance, and advocacy. Provides information on lead abatement and legislation.

Environmental Defense Fund

5655 College Avenue, Suite 304
Oakland CA 94618

Shopper's Guide: What You Should Know About Lead in China Dishes. *A consumer's guide which also provides manufacturers and potentially safer alternatives.*

American College for Advancement in Medicine

23121 Verdugo Drive, Suite 204
Laguna Hills CA 92653
(800)532-3688
(714)583-7666
(714)455-9679 Fax

Provides physician referral for chelation therapy.

Feingold Association of the United States

P.O. Box 6550
Alexandria VA 22306
(703)768-3287

Dietary consultation and programs for helping attention deficit disorder children without using drugs.

Mothers and Others for a Livable Planet

P.O. Box 98111
Washington DC 20077
(202)783-7800

Reading list and newsletter to help reduce exposure to pesticides.

National Safety Council, National Lead Information Center

(800)532-3394
A toll-free hotline in English or Spanish that provides information on protecting children from lead poisoning.

Practical Allergy Research Foundation

P.O. Box 60
Buffalo NY 14223
(800)787-8780

Physician referrals for children. Reference materials on children's chemical and food sensitivity and related behavioral problems. Offers a video, "Environmentally Sick Schools."

20. DON'T SWEAT IT . . . YES, DO!

"The inevitable question surfaces: should we ever have got to the stage where we have to decontaminate . . . people? However you answer the question, the fact remains that we are no longer talking simply of wildlife, we are talking about us. When *Silent Spring* burst on a largely unsuspecting world, we were talking about the reproductive failures of animals and birds. Today we know that our sperm, our eggs, our embryos and our children are also in the front line."

—John Elkington[1]

Henry sweats too much. He sweats at work. He sweats in the car. He sweats on a date—his last girlfriend wore a rain slicker. Gillette once offered Henry ten thousand dollars to spend three weeks as a test subject in their antiperspirant development lab. The only time Henry looks normal is at the gym. So why is he smiling? Henry might be about the least toxic guy on Earth.

The pollution of the human body has been going on quietly for decades. Small amounts of synthetic, manmade pesticides, drugs, and other pollutants have found their way into soil, water, air, crops, animals, and *you*.[2] Nature has no way of breaking these down. They accumulate in your fat. We all have fat. It's not just on our backside or midriff bulge. You don't have to be out of shape to have fat in your body, it's part of our internal organs, it coats our nervous system, and makes up much of our brains. The EPA took human fat samples from people across the country and found virtually everyone has measurable amounts of toxins in their fat.[3] Common sense says the higher your internal dose, the higher your risk.

Did You Know:

- If these poisons stayed in your fat, there might be less reason for concern. However, these chemicals move from the fat into the bloodstream when you are under physical stress.
- "The fact that the average suburbanite is not instantly stricken has little meaning. The toxins may sleep long in the body, to become manifest months or even years later in an obscure disorder almost impossible to trace to its origins."[4]
- Your body contains as many as one hundred seventy-seven different kinds of organochlorines.[5]

- The largest excretory organ in the human body is the skin. The skin has two excretion pathways: oil glands (sebum) and water glands (sweat). The Mt. Sinai School of Medicine and other researchers have found chemicals and medical and illegal drugs are excreted through skin oil and sweat.[6,7,8]
- The Hubbard detoxification program was developed in the 1970s primarily to assist recovering drug addicts by flushing out drug and chemical residues. The program has since undergone some ten independent scientific studies documenting the program's safety and effectiveness for lowering body burdens of industrial chemicals and pesticides.[9,10,11,12,13,14,15,16,17,18,19]

SYMPTOM IMPROVEMENT AFTER DETOXIFICATION[20]

Symptom	Symptoms Before Detoxification (percent)	Symptoms After Detoxification (percent)
Rash	18	4
Acne	16	4
Weakness	16	4
Incoordination	7	0
Dizziness	18	2
Fatigue	79	5
Nervousness	14	4
Disorientation	11	0
Headaches	40	9
Joint pain	5	0
Muscle pain	42	5

SIMPLE THINGS TO DO

- If you have a concern about toxic buildup, ask your doctor to test for toxins in your body (see Chapter 17).
- Exercise frequently and *really* sweat.
- Insure your diet is rich in "phytomins," antioxidants, and other protectants (see Chapter 18).
- Supervised detoxification programs are available.

RESOURCES

Bridge Publications
4751 Fountain Avenue
Los Angeles CA 90029
(800)722-1733

A self-help video and manual that provides information required to do a detoxification program on your own.

Doctor Ronald Maugeri
Rittenhouse Health Care Systems
1930 Chestnut St.
Philadelphia PA 19103
(215)563-2221

Supervised detoxification.

David Root, M.D.
HealthMed
5501 Power Inn Road, Suite 140
Sacramento CA 95820
(916)924-8060

Supervised detoxification.

21. LOOK WHO'S COMING

Although we can't control nature and genetics has a huge impact, many birth defects are preventable. We've all heard about the impact of substances on the fetus (think of all those medications labeled with "If you are pregnant consult your doctor before taking this product") and we've seen the warning labels on alcohol. What most people don't know is prevention of birth defects begins *before* conception. So if you're thinking about having a baby think about these questions. Do you guys booze? Do you use drugs? Are you around pesticides or other chemicals at work or in the home? What you eat, drink, and do and the environment around you can have an effect not only on your ability to conceive but on your kid once you are pregnant. So get ready. Here comes junior.

DID YOU KNOW:

- Seven percent of children in the United States are born with birth defects that are immediately apparent or appear later in life.
- The occurrence of birth defects has increased dramatically in recent years. Between 1970 and 1985, eighteen of the twenty-seven most common birth defects increased. Some went up as much as seventeen hundred percent.[1]
- A fifty-percent reduction in birth defect rates could be achieved through a combination of improved diet and toxic exposure reduction.[2]
- A woman's diet and her lifestyle are important during pregnancy and the months before pregnancy. A *pre*-pregnancy health program will dramatically reduce risks of miscarriage and birth defects.[3,4,5,6]
- In the United Kingdom, women following a prepregnancy health program have an overall birth defect rate of less than one percent, compared to the five to seven percent rate for women on no program in the United States and England.[7]
- Dieting immediately before and during pregnancy increases your baby's chances of having birth defects and susceptibility to diseases including anemia, heart and lung problems, as well as raising the risk of premature birth and lowered birth weight.[8]
- A few studies have correlated high caffeine consumption to an increased risk of miscarriage and infertility.[9,10] Caffeine readily passes to the unborn.[11] Coffee and caffeinated drinks affect nutritional status, reducing vitamins and minerals.[12] Caffeine is in many soft drinks, hot chocolates, and teas.
- Medical drugs, sometimes given to pregnant women to take, are associated with birth defects. Forty-five percent of all pregnant

women in five Connecticut hospitals received prescription drugs, such as antidepressants or water pills, that contributed about thirteen percent to the total birth defect rate.[13] Street drugs can do the same or far worse.

- Eating cured meats such as hot dogs, salami, bacon, and smoked fish is risky at all times for both men and women. These contain nitrite that interacts with other chemicals in the food itself or in the stomach to form potent cancer-causing chemicals.[14] Men's consumption of hot dogs is associated with an increased risk of leukemia for the children they father.[15] A mother eating cured meats during pregnancy appears to increase her child's risk of brain cancer.[16,17,18,19]

- Prepregnancy exposure to pesticides increases your baby's risk of being born with a birth defect or later contracting cancer (see Chapters 10 and 24).[20]

- Radiation exposure to the mother's egg can cause cell damage, leading to birth defects or an increased risk of childhood cancer.

- Unfiltered and polluted tap water is strongly associated with an increased risk of birth defects.[21,22,23]

- Men also need to be aware. "There is growing evidence that human sperm can provide a direct route into the womb for many of our most dangerous pollutants. The sperm may yet prove to be the Trojan horse of reproductive toxicology."[24] Some believe eighty percent of birth defects stem from the father's sperm.[25]

- A study of sperm quality among college students found traces of the toxic chemical that is used as a flame retardant in foam-filled furniture such as mattresses. Other chemicals found included PCBs, shown to cause human birth defects; DDT, which causes reproductive toxicity; and benzene, which causes cancer. In total, some twenty different chemicals with potential adverse effects on sperm quality and production were found. Twenty-three percent of those tested had sperm counts that were so low, they were probably sterile.[26] Men's low sperm counts also cause birth defects.[27]

- Men who smoke tend to father children with lower birth weights and who are more likely to die young.[28]

- Men involved in jobs with toxic chemicals suffer sperm cell damage, or bring home residues and dust.[29,30,31,32,33]

SIMPLE THINGS TO DO

Diet

- Mom should not diet or embark on a weight-loss program prior to or during pregnancy.
- Organically grown foods are important for both mom and dad in their diet for two reasons: greater nutritional value and absence of pesticides that can cause birth defects and cancer (see Chapter 24).
- Emphasize a diet rich in leafy, dark green vegetables such as collards, kale, and mustard greens, which are rich in vitamins and minerals. Eat a colorful selection of fresh fruits, other vegetables, and whole grains.
- If your diet does not supply enough of the basic nutrients, many doctors recommend supplementing with vitamins and minerals, especially folic acid.[34,35,36]

Foods to Avoid

See also Chapter 32

- Be careful about your seafood choices. Swordfish, bluefish, lake trout, whitefish, and Maine and Massachusetts lobster should definitely be avoided by women of childbearing age, due to contamination with reproductive toxins such as mercury and PCBs. A general rule of thumb: avoid freshwater fish, especially those from the nation's inland waterways.[37] (See Chapter 25).
- Limit consumption of cured meats.
- Cut down on coffee to no more than two cups daily. Cut down or eliminate soda drinks and caffeinated tea.

Environmental Considerations

- Don't use home and garden pesticides.
- Avoid X-rays unless absolutely necessary. If women must un-

dergo X-rays, insist that the technician place a lead apron over the area around the ovaries.
- Don't scrape or sand old paint, as this can cause lead dust.
- Avoid hair dye use even before conception (see Chapter 42).
- On the job, men and women should know what chemicals they are using and avoid exposure if they intend to have children. Employers supply material safety data sheets (MSDSs) that provide information on the toxicity of chemicals to which workers are exposed. Refer to books on workplace chemicals.
- Have your tap water tested for contamination with lead, industrial solvents, pesticides, and other pollutants. If poisons are present, filter your water or use a safer source (see Chapter 27).

Prescription, Illegal, and Recreational Drugs

- Stop smoking. Don't drink alcohol. Don't use any illegal street drugs. All these toxins go straight to the unborn.
- Stop using over-the-counter or prescription drugs at least three months prior to pregnancy, as it often takes several months for birth defect-causing drugs such as the acne drug, Accutane, to clear from your body. (Before stopping a prescription medication abruptly, discuss this with your doctor.)
- If you must use a medication, consult your doctor *and* the *Physicians' Desk Reference* to learn of any potential harm during pregnancy.

A Sperm Improvement Plan

Men, quit smoking. Supplemental vitamin C at doses as low as a thousand milligrams have helped couples to become pregnant. A study showed that about one hundred twenty milligrams of zinc sulfate on a twice-daily basis increased the sperm count in thirty-seven males with low sperm counts and infertility for over five years. One report noted that one hundred seventy-eight men with low sperm counts were given four grams daily of the amino acid L-arginine, and that one hundred eleven had marked improvement and twenty-one moderate improvement. Men who eat organic foods have sperm counts that are about twice as high as men who don't (see Chapter 30).

RESOURCES

National Institute of Environmental Health and Safety (NIEHS)
Enviro-Health Clearinghouse
100 Capitola Drive, Suite 108
Durham NC 27713
(800)643-4794

Enviro-Health is a NIEHS clearinghouse that functions as an easily accessible, free source of information on environmental health effects, including industrial chemicals. Use the toll-free number for information.

Perinatal Health, Inc.
7777 Greenback Lane, Suite 205
Citrus Heights CA 95610
(916)725-4035

A woman who wants further help on getting ready for pregnancy should contact and order a computer-scored questionnaire, called the Before Pregnancy Health Inventory. After completion, she will receive a custom twenty- to thirty-page guide to help determine which changes to make to reduce her child's risk of birth defects.

Part III

DIET FOR A NEW LIFE

———————— 🐟 ————————

22. YOU ARE WHAT YOU EAT—

AND THEN SOME

When Harry was a little boy he'd put just about anything in his mouth: snails, nails, worms, and dog fur balls. His mother was convinced he was a goat in a past life. Harry's a mature adult now, the respected superintendent of a local refinery, and a far more discriminating connoisseur. He chases down his breakfast bacon and eggs with two quarter pounders with cheese for lunch and tops it off with pepperoni pizza for dinner. Harry smiles, remembering his mom's warning, "You are what you eat, son." He's not mooing or oinking yet. But Harry hasn't heard the true story of Marie.

Marie's Story

Marie (a pseudonym) was a simple woman from the village of Semic in the former Yugoslavia. Like most of the villagers, her family had their own vegetable garden, chickens, goats, and cows. They drew their water from a local well. In hard economic times, they had to ensure they had enough food. Marie worked at the one factory in the village. Almost everybody worked there. The factory made electrical devices. Her job was to stand on a production line and inspect electric transformers by hand. If they leaked, she threw them in a reject bin; if not, they passed on down the line. Marie started getting sick. Her skin broke out with acne so large it scarred her body. Her stomach and joints swelled. She was always tired. Her breasts continually discharged a bluish-green liquid. The village doctor didn't know how to treat her. Finally, a doctor from the University of Ljubljana ran tests. Her liver was enlarged, and her immune system was dangerously damaged.

The doctor was smart. He asked about her job. He discovered the oil used in the electrical devices she inspected contained a deadly toxin, PCBs. He knew PCBs could be absorbed through the skin. She never was given protective gloves. He tested and found her tissue levels of PCBs were one hundred times higher than average in unexposed persons. The breast discharge was seven hundred times higher than her tissue levels. Even more chilling, the entire village, its water, its people, its animals, and its food sources were all contaminated with PCB wastes dumped by the factory for years.[1] In addition to working with these chemicals, Marie had been eating and drinking them for years.

Marie went through detoxification (see Chapter 20), the PCBs were reduced, and her symptoms went away. But what Marie will never forget, and neither should Harry, is that we are the chemicals we eat, drink, and breathe.[2]

23. SAVE YOUR WAISTLINE WHILE POISONS

MISS THE MARK

"High cholesterol levels are like red flags warning us that the body is storing too many toxins."

—JOSEPH WEISSMAN, M.D.[1]

We hear so much about cholesterol *this* and fat *that*. It's everywhere—CNN, *Good Morning America*. That's just what you want to hear over morning coffee—how your arteries are so clogged you need a physician-turned-Roto-Rooter-man to augur them out. At night, you start dreaming . . . visions of a miniature Al Bundy with a jackhammer working his way down the carotid artery in your neck. We've become so fixated on cholesterol and fat, we forget that they are an essential part of the diet. They provide the raw materials for many key functions of your body.[2,3] In fact, if your diet is too low in fats and cholesterol, you may be at increased risk of depression.[4] Not to mention that if you don't eat enough of them, your joints will stiffen, your glands will shrink, and you will lose your sexual desire.

But, on the other hand, there are "good fats" such as olive oil and flax oil, and there are "bad fats" such as those found in beef and dairy products and used in margarine. No doubt, eating less of the bad fats and more of the good ones is smart. But what would you think if someone told you, in the case of cancer, it may not be the fat at all. It's true, but before you run out and buy two Big Macs and pig out, get the facts.

Animal fat has much higher concentrations of toxins than many fruits, vegetables, and grains.[5,6,7] Evidence from humans and experimental animals makes it clear that toxins in animal fat, not just the fat, cause cancer.[8,9] Eating lower on the food chain, more fruits and vegetables and grains, is not only good for your waistline and your heart—it will reduce your cancer risk.

Nature's Revenge

Many industrial chemicals and pesticides that are sprayed on crops, dumped into oceans and streams, spewed into the sky, or that contaminate the soil, last for decades. They go into the fish, chickens, pigs, and cows. Since animals don't digest them, they build up in their fat.[10] They show up in our butter, milk, cheese, bacon, and hamburgers. Because man is at the top end of the food chain, we are the final garbage dump.[11]

DID YOU KNOW:

- A typical beef/pork hot dog in the United States contains seven cancer-causing pesticides in every bite. Heavy hot dog diets have been linked to increased cancers in children.
- A typical quarter-pound burger contains three cancer-causing pesticides in every bite.
- Dieldrin, found in much of the beef sold in supermarkets, causes cancer.[12]
- The primary source of dioxin and nuclear radiation contamination in humans is from beef and dairy products.[13,14]

SIMPLE THINGS TO DO

- Eat low on the food chain. Choose fruits, vegetables, and grains over meat.
- Limit your intake of dairy products.
- When your kids have a hot dog or burger, substitute turkey or chicken for beef or pork.
- Make red meat the exception in your diet, not the rule. And when you do eat red meat, eat lean.
- Sources of good fats include olive and flax oils, as well as seafood.

24. EAT IT—*ORGANIC*

"Propelled by dynamic growth of more than 22 percent in 1994, the organic industry smashed through the $2 billion sales barrier, continuing its powerful climb into the upper strata of high-growth trade."

—*Natural Foods Merchandiser,*
June 1995[1]

All right, if we mention organic foods, you're probably thinking of hippies in Birkenstock sandals, funky communes out in the country, and love-ins at the park. It also could be you're thinking of worms in your apples, stunted crooked carrots, and shrunken heads of lettuce. If that's where some people are at, we've got news for them: They're caught in a time warp!

Today organic foods are a leading American growth industry, and the "hippies" are now yuppies driving brand new BMWs.

Gallo Vineyards, once the archrival of Cesar Chavez and the United Farm Workers, is now the largest organic farmer in the United States.[2]

Wake up to the new organic agriculture!

Did You Know:

- Instead of using powerful toxic pesticides that persist for months to decades in the environment, organic farmers use beneficial insects or other substances that quickly break down and that are virtually harmless, both to the environment and the consumers of the produce. The big bonus is that organic farmers' methods do not pollute drinking water supplies, threaten wildlife, or endanger the health of farmers, farm workers, and YOU.
- Organically grown foods contain significantly higher amounts of important trace elements, needed for optimum health, than foods grown conventionally with pesticides.[3]
- Organic foods have smaller amounts of toxic metals such as aluminum, lead, and mercury.[4]
- Organic meat and poultry, particularly beef, is free from residues of hormone implants and other cancer-causing animal drugs (see Chapters 30 and 31).
- Organic dairy products are virtually free of antibiotics and other animal drugs such as bovine growth hormone (see Chapter 37).
- *More sex. Better sex.* Organic farmers and others who eat foods grown without pesticides have "an unexpectedly high sperm density," in spite of having sex more frequently.[5] Men in this study who consumed organic foods, in fact, had *twice* the sperm count of those who didn't.

- In a study with rabbits, infant survival rate was higher in the group fed organic diets.[6]
- *What goes around comes around.* Farmers who spray pesticides have a higher cancer risk.[7,8,9,10]
- Nowadays one in three shoppers seeks out organically grown fruits and vegetables.[11]
- A study in California found that of nearly three hundred fifty samples of organically grown produce, only three percent had any detectable pesticide residues.[12] Roughly fifty to seventy-five percent of chemically grown foods are contaminated with one or more pesticide residues, including those that cause cancer, birth defects, and nervous or immune system damage.[13,14,15,16]

SIMPLE THINGS TO DO

- When shopping for organic foods, make sure a label is on the packaging or attached to the food bin stating the food is certified organic by any of several internationally recognized groups: California Certified Organic Farmers (CCOF), Farm Verified Organic (FVO), Organic Crop Improvement Association (OCIA), Organic Foods Production Association of North America (OFPANA), Oregon Tilth, and Washington Tilth.
- If food isn't certified, it still may be organic, if you shop farmer's markets.
- Organic produce must be handled and stored properly. Immediately refrigerate fresh produce. Fruits, such as apples and oranges, should be refrigerated, not left on the counter. Organic grain products should always be stored in tightly sealed containers.

RESOURCES

Americans for Safe Food
1875 Connecticut Avenue N.W., Suite 300
Washington DC 20009-5728
(202)332-9110

Guide to mail order organic food.

Coleman Natural Meats

5140 Race Court, Unit 4
Denver CO 80216
(303)297-9393

Organically raised beef available at stores nationwide.

Mothers and Others

40 West 20th Street
New York New York 10011
(212)242-0010

For $1.00, provides a Mother's Milk List *that lists brand names, supermarkets, dairies, and distributors that offer products from cows that have not been treated with synthetic bovine growth hormone (rBGH).*

Horizon Organic Dairy

P.O. 17577
Boulder CO 80308
(303)530-2711

Organic dairy products available at stores nationwide.

Royal Blue Organics

P.O. Box 21123
Eugene OR 97402
(503)689-1836
(800)392-0117

Organic coffee by mail.

25. SOMETHING FISHY

"At its best, seafood is as safe as any organic fruit or vegetable. . . . At its worst, seafood is the most dangerous source of powerful cancer-causing chemicals in our diet."

—*DIET FOR A POISONED PLANET*[1]

Seafood is a rich source of low-fat protein, vitamins, and minerals. Its regular consumption, as part of an overall heart-healthy diet, rich in fresh fruits, vegetables, whole grains, and olive oil, offers protection against heart disease.[2,3,4,5,6,7] Not surprisingly, many Americans are making the switch from red meat to seafood. However, they may be jumping from the fatty frying pan into the toxic fire.[8]

Not Just Another Fish Story

Renee Jones loved fishing with her children at Venice Pier in Los Angeles. She and her children would often spend the weekend there, catching local perch and halibut, frying them up, and having a picnic. It was a nice way to spend the weekend.

Renee (not her real name) was part of a group of subjects whose blood serum was being analyzed by researchers for pollution levels resulting from eating locally caught food. The level of DDT in her blood was thirteen times higher than the average level of DDT in the blood of Americans today. She wasn't alone. The researchers discovered many other fish-eaters had elevated concentrations of DDT and PCBs. The common link between them all was frequent consumption of fish from polluted Santa Monica Bay.[9]

DID YOU KNOW:

- More than two thousand advisories have been issued nationwide, warning against eating contaminated seafood.[10]
- The National Academy of Sciences conservatively concluded that for every one million seafood consumers in the country seventy-five will develop cancer from pollutants in their seafood.[11]
- Studies show high body burdens of pesticides and industrial chemicals, including those found in seafood, are associated with an increased risk of cancer.[12,13,14,15,16] Seafood alone is not the cause of these cancers. But toxic seafood could be part of an overall toxic diet.
- Mercury causes birth defects (see Chapter 21). Recent evidence indicates it may be a cause of heart disease and Parkinson's disease (see Chapter 41). A high intake of mercury from freshwater fish and consequent accumulation of mercury in the body are associated with an excess risk of heart disease and deaths from coronary heart disease, including stroke.[17] Elevated blood mercury levels are tied to risk of Parkinson's disease.[18]
- Babies born to women who regularly eat PCB-contaminated fish suffer subtle birth defects, including smaller birth weight and nerve damage, that not only persist as they grow up but become the cause of obvious mental handicaps. The mothers ate only a few polluted meals a month.[19,20,21,22]
- Safe seafood, such as wild Pacific salmon, when it is safe, is an important food in the diet because of its content of docosahexaenoic acid (DHA) which helps lower risk of heart disease and also may counteract depression.[23]

SIMPLE THINGS TO DO

You won't get this information at your local seafood shop, supermarket, or restaurant, so we've reviewed FDA monitoring files obtained through the Freedom of Information Act to tell you which fish are safe (green); which are deserving of caution (yellow); and which are too dangerous to eat (red). While pollution levels in fish can vary by season and location, these are good guidelines to follow.

Green Light (Safest)

These fish on the average have the smallest concentrations of industrial pollutants and pesticides and should be the mainstays of your seafood menu.

Abalone

Arctic char

Crab (from California, Georgia, Argentina, China, or Korea)

Dungeness crab

Imitation crab

Crawfish

Grouper

Haddock

Halibut (from Alaska or Iceland)

Mahimahi

Orange roughy

Pacific salmon (wild)

Pollock

Red snapper

Sea bass

Shrimp, domestic and imported, is virtually pollution free. Because of the possible use of banned antibiotics in foreign farm-raised shrimp, choose United States–harvested shrimp.

Spiny lobster (from Australia, New Zealand, or California)

Squid (calamari)

Talapia

Tuna (generally safe, at times may contain trace amounts of mercury, which is particularly dangerous to pregnant women and their unborn babies. Limit to a few times a month.)

Wahoo

Whiting

Yellowtail

Yellow Light (Proceed With Caution)

Fish in this category tend to contain significantly higher amounts of contaminants than those under the green light heading. Eat seldom.

Bonito (from California)
Crab (from Chesapeake Bay)
Ocean perch (from California)
Rainbow trout (farm-raised)
Rock cod (from California)
Sea trout (from New Jersey)
Thresher shark
Whitefish

Red Light (Stop!)

These fish don't belong in your shopping cart. According to government reports, they can contain the highest concentrations of a wide range of carcinogens including benzene hexachloride, chlordane, DDT, dieldrin, dioxin, endrin, heptachlor, pentachlorophenol, and toxaphene. Toss them back!

Black cod (also sold as California black cod, butterfish, and sablefish)

Bluefish

Buffalo fish

Carp

Catfish (including farm-raised)

Chub

Cod (do not eat if from California and the Pacific northwest; from elsewhere it's OK.)

Coho salmon (do not eat if from the Great Lakes; from elsewhere it's OK.)

Lobster (do not eat if from Maine and Massachusetts; from elsewhere it's OK.)

Swordfish

Shellfish Alert

Don't eat raw shellfish. They can be contaminated with microorganisms, some naturally occurring, others due to pollution. Especially vulnerable are people with weakened immune systems due to cancer, AIDS, and liver disease, as well as the elderly and children under the age of two.[24] Steamed and cooked shellfish are safer.

26. How Sweet It Isn't

"It is interesting to note that the first experiments done to test the safety of aspartame before its final approval in 1981 disclosed a high incidence of brain tumors in animals fed Nutrasweet. In fact, this study was done by the manufacturer of Nutrasweet, G. D. Searle."

—Russell Blaylock, M.D.
Excitotoxins[1]

Joe and Sally are taking their son, Tommy, to the movies—the fourteenth time they're seeing *Lion King*. Joe orders a diet soda and Tommy a no-sugar Popsicle, both with Nutrasweet; Sally gets a cup of coffee with lowfat milk and Equal—so she can stay awake. They're on diets. They take their seats, proud they resisted the buttered popcorn and Jujubes. The only problem is that Sally needs a shoehorn to fit in her seat, Joe's gut hangs out so far that when he stands to let people by they get stuck in the aisle, and Tommy's so pudgy that dad was charged for *two* tickets. They've sworn off sugar for the past three months but they're still FAT!

It's estimated that more than one hundred fifty million Americans use artificial sweeteners.[2] We're constantly bombarded with propaganda about how important it is to be thin. While TV commercials and Cher pave the yellow brick road to being thin with artificial sweeteners, there is evidence that says exactly the opposite is true! Americans are fatter than ever, and they use more no-calorie artificial sweeteners nowadays than ever before.

Did You Know:

• In 1975 the average American's consumption of artificial sweeteners was the equivalent of six pounds of sugar. In 1984 it was sixteen pounds. Did this reduce the total amount of *actual* sugar consumed? No! It went from one hundred eighteen pounds per person in 1975 to one hundred twenty-six pounds in 1984. People ate MORE sugar![3]

- There is little proof that artificial sweeteners are useful for weight loss.[4,5,6,7]
- When experimental animals were given artificial sweeteners in their drinking water, they ate more and became fatter. Only when the artificial sweetener was given in massive enough dosages to make the food taste bad did the animals eat less.
- More than ten thousand people have reported side effects using aspartame.[8]
- The most common complaints from people using aspartame are headaches, blurred vision, and seizures.[9,10]
- Aspartame is also linked to dry eyes, memory loss, and depression.[11]
- Aspartame turns into four chemicals in your body: methanol, formaldehyde, aspartic acid, and phenylalanine. These chemicals have been associated with headaches, seizures, blurred vision, muscular pains, cancer, nerve damage, brain lesions, and birth defects.[12,13]
- Not only don't you lose weight—you may be damaging your brain. Stupid and fat? No, thank you!
- Children are at greater risk from artificial sweeteners because, pound for pound, they eat more than adults and their nervous systems are still not fully developed.

Nutragate

An investigation of the FDA approval process for Nutrasweet found that the administration trivialized studies showing increased brain cancer in animals. FDA employees or consultants involved in the approval were later discovered working for the company that made aspartame.[14,15]

SIMPLE THINGS TO DO

- Avoid artificial sweeteners. You're better off using black-strap molasses, honey, or maple syrup. Even a teeny bit of sugar is better than the synthetic stuff.
- Check labels. You'll find aspartame in Popsicles, ice cream, soft drinks, Jell-O, candy, gum, and many other packaged foods.
- Try an apple or an orange. Fruits will satisfy most urges for sweets. It really works!
- Eat cereals, sodas, and cookies sweetened with fruit juice.

27. WATER, WATER EVERYWHERE AND NOT A DROP TO DRINK

"We haven't the faintest idea how to test multiple chemicals. We don't know how to test two, let alone four, five, or ten. I doubt that any water tested is going to have only one pesticide or only one chemical. It is going to have a whole host."

—VERNON N. HOUK, M.D.[1]

At least one hundred twenty-one thousand miles of rivers and streams have been polluted by agricultural and industrial pollution.[2] Anybody getting thirsty?

In 1990 in the United States, toxic discharges into surface waters amounted to one hundred ninety-seven million pounds, including more than two and a half million pounds of carcinogens.[3] Thirsty yet?

Some forty-three percent of the nation's community water systems are in violation of federal safe drinking water laws.[4] More than twenty-three million of us are slurping down fecal matter, radiation, industrial chemicals, and other "taste enhancers."[5]

Are you running for the bottled water?

DID YOU KNOW:

- The Centers for Disease Control (CDC) reports that more than nine hundred thousand people become sick in the United States annually due to bacterial contamination of drinking water.[6]

- *Ban the squirt gun, too.* Chlorination of drinking water is an important public health measure to eliminate deadly bacteria. Yet, in spite of its critical importance, chlorination poses its own set of health concerns. One commonly occurring type of drinking water contaminant, trihalomethanes, produced when polluted water is disinfected with chlorine, is responsible for nearly eleven thousand bladder and rectal cancers annually.[7] "This is twice as many people as are killed in fires and more than are killed by handguns."[8]

- Arsenic, often thought of as rat poison, is a common drinking water contaminant.[9,10]

- More than forty-nine million people drink water that is significantly radioactive.[11,12]

- In California alone, from Sacramento to Los Angeles, some one million people have consumed water with detectable concentrations of a toxic chemical that mimics the natural human hormone estrogen.[13] "More than 20 large public systems, including the water supply for Disneyland, that bastion of childhood innocence and fantasy, have been tainted."[14] *Say it ain't so, Mickey.*

- A recent sampling of tap water in the Midwest, Maryland, and Louisiana found that twenty-eight of twenty-nine cities' drinking water contained atrazine, a weed killer used on corn and associated with human ovarian cancer.[15]

- Drinking water contaminated with industrial chemicals has been shown to increase the risk of leukemia among New Jersey women.[16]

- Lead is one of the most dangerous drinking water contaminants (see Chapter 19). The relationship between lead levels in teeth

and classroom performance was investigated in one hundred fifty-eight schoolchildren. Those with high lead levels scored significantly lower on learning tests.[17]
- Consumption of unfiltered or polluted tap water is associated with miscarriages and birth defects.[18,19]
- Women who drink filtered water have a lower than normal risk of adverse pregnancy outcome.[20]

Gimme Five, Dude

Drinking water standards are the weakest of all federal environmental regulations. There are five good reasons for this:

1. The testers look at each chemical and set limits on them individually. They never test for the effect of a combination of chemicals, the way they really occur in drinking water.
2. Many chemical contaminants break down in water. Their breakdown products may be as toxic as the originals. The EPA does not take this into account when setting safe drinking water standards.
3. The EPA ignores seasonal differences. During certain times of the year, farmers bomb their crops with heavy applications of pesticides. During these periods, millions of people drink water contaminated at levels above EPA health standards.[21]
4. EPA does not account for increased risks to the fetus, infants, and children.
5. EPA standards are largely based on preventing cancer. They ignore danger to the immune and nervous systems. These may be injured by doses that current standards consider safe.[22]

SIMPLE THINGS TO DO

- Call or write your drinking water supplier. Request its most recent report on what is in your drinking water. Such a report should include industrial chemicals, metals, chlorination by-products, pesticides, radioactivity, and bacteria. If your water contains any of these, consider having it filtered.

- *Don't be penny wise and gallon foolish.* Test your water personally. Such tests may cost up to two hundred dollars, but they provide useful information and personal protection. They are a small investment in prevention, especially compared to possible medical bills.

It's a Lead-Pipe Cinch

Watch out for lead contamination. The use of lead water mains and service connections is common in many older cities. Home piping was made of lead until about 1930, and lead solder has been used to join copper pipes since at least 1949.[23]

Such pipes should be replaced with stainless steel or copper. Have your plumber remove any lead-soldered connections and replace them with longer lengths of pipe and fewer connections, using silver solder.

- Filter your water with a system combining activated carbon and an ultra filtration process known as reverse osmosis. These units fit under the sink and are available for a few hundred dollars. These might provide you with the cleanest water you can drink and save you a lot of money on bottled water.
- Switching to bottled water when you have contaminated tap water—and *mucho* bucks—makes sense if you don't filter your water. But bottled water could be as contaminated as tap water.[24,25,26,27]
- If you must drink unfiltered water from the tap, allow the water to run for a minute before using. This reduces the level of lead in the water.
- Consider the use of a Brita-style pitcher water filter.

RESOURCES

Water Filters

National Sanitation Foundation
3475 Plymouth Road
P.O. Box 1468
Ann Arbor MI 48106
(313)769-8010

Certifiers of water filters.

Water Testing

National Testing Laboratories
6151 Wilson Mills Road
Cleveland OH 44143
(800)458-3330
(216)449-2525

Water testing.

Suburban Water Testing Laboratories
4600 Kutztown Road
Temple PA 19560
(800)433-6595
(215)929-3666

Water testing.

General Information

EPA Drinking Water Information Hot Line
(800)426-4791
(800)424-LEAD

Water Quality Association
4151 Naperville Road
Lisle IL 60532

Information on water quality problems and filters.

28. YOU MAKE ME SO EXCITED . . .

"What if someone were to tell you that a chemical added to food could cause brain damage in your children, so that in later years they have learning or emotional difficulties? The only study being conducted on the long-term effects of excitotoxins is on us."

—RUSSELL BLAYLOCK, M.D.[1]

You're on a blind date, and it's a dog. But as you jam down the chips, dip, and sodas your date starts looking better and better—in spite of the buck-teeth, braces, and about a million zits. It's not that you're horny, or even hard up. It's not the "great conversation" either: your date barely mumbles an occasional grunt.

Maybe it's the food.

Your meal could be loaded with excitotoxins.

Sound scary? It is. Sound complex? It isn't. An excitotoxin is a specific type of amino acid. While all amino acids play an essential role in health as building blocks of proteins, the trouble comes when certain amino acids, used as food additives, are added to the food supply in uncontrolled amounts. When eaten in excess by vulnerable individuals, including babies and children, excitotoxins overexcite the nervous system, causing cells to die.

DID YOU KNOW:

• The brain has a protective outer covering, the blood-brain barrier, that limits the amount of toxins that enter. However, psychiatric drugs, low blood sugar, crash diets, fevers, exposure to lead, viruses, head injuries, and high blood pressure weaken or temporarily break down the blood-brain barrier.

- The three largest sources of excitotoxins in the diet are the additives monosodium glutamate (MSG), hydrolyzed vegetable protein (HVP), and aspartame (Nutrasweet or Equal). These contain the amino acids aspartate, glutamate, and phenylalanine, which are derived from a normal diet and are essential at lower levels but become excitotoxins when consumed in largely uncontrolled excessive amounts.
- MSG is an artificial taste enhancer added to bland food to make it taste better. It's added to soups, gravies, chips, low-fat foods, fast foods, ready-made dinners, and canned goods.
- HVP is used to create a beefy taste in hot dogs, soups, and barbecue sauces, as well as to add a creamy texture to processed foods ranging from frozen dinners to nondairy creamers. It is made by boiling vegetables in sulfuric acid, neutralizing the soup with caustic soda, and drying it to a brown sludge. Sounds appetizing, doesn't it?
- A child's brain is much more sensitive to excitotoxins than an adult's.[2,3,4]
- Scientific evidence indicates MSG could cause brain damage in newborns.[5,6,7]
- A child eating soup with MSG and a diet soda with aspartame raises his blood level of excitotoxins six times higher than necessary to cause brain damage in experimental animals.[8] The combined effect of MSG and aspartame is more toxic to the brain than either would be individually.
- Excitotoxins in a child's diet have been linked to behavioral problems, including hyperactivity, learning disabilities, dyslexia, rage, and violence, as well as obesity, stunted growth, headaches, and seizures.[9]
- A lifetime consumption of excitotoxins is thought by some to contribute to, or hasten the onset of, brain disorders such as Alzheimer's disease, Parkinson's disease, and Huntington's disease.[10,11,12,13]

When I Call Your Name . . .

Additives that always contain MSG:
Hydrolyzed vegetable protein
Hydrolyzed protein
Hydrolyzed plant protein
Sodium caseinate
Calcium caseinate
Yeast extract
Textured protein
Autolyzed yeast
Hydrolyzed oat flour

SIMPLE THINGS TO DO

- Avoid processed and packaged foods with labels that list MSG or HVP.
- Drink natural juices or soda sweetened with fruit juice.
- Don't drink diet sodas with aspartame or saccharin.
- Avoid tranquilizers, stimulants, and psychiatric drugs.
- Pregnant women and people with high blood pressure, previous excess exposure to toxic chemicals, nutritional deficiencies, and stress should avoid excitotoxins.

RESOURCES

No MSG
P.O. Box 367
Santa Fe NM 87504

Provides information on MSG.

Citizens Commission on Human Rights
6362 Hollywood Blvd., Suite B
Los Angeles CA 90028
(213)467-4242

Provides information on drug side effects and nondrug alternatives for hyperactive children.

29. GROW YOUR OWN

More than 30 million Americans have gardens.

Willis has been searching for a parking spot at the supermarket for half an hour. Finally he spots a woman getting into her car. He waits. What's she doing reading *War and Peace*? Five cars back up behind him angrily honking their horns. Finally she backs out, but a red Porsche darts in and steals "his" spot. Willis jumps out of his car ready to yell in the driver's face when he discovers that it is a very attractive woman. She says, "Thank you, dear," which melts Willis and sends him back to his car to look for another spot. With no spaces left and without a twinge of guilt Willis parks in a handicapped spot and fakes a limp as he goes past the security guard. The supermarket never ceases to amaze Willis. There's a lady on the end of one aisle with a hotplate on a table stuffing smelly cheese on top of stale melba toast into anyone hungry or dumb enough to open their mouths. There are video games, pots and pans, lottery tickets, a gourmet section, a wine section, a gourmet wine section, an espresso bar, forty checkers, five security guards, and assistant managers by the dozens.

Willis sighs and gets on the "10 items or less" line behind twelve people who have an average of fifteen items each and who are all trying to read the tabloids without looking like they are trying to. Finally, Willis pays the checker $1.95 for a head of lettuce and walks out to the parking lot to discover that his car has been towed. Willis could spare himself some aggravation, save his money, and save his health if he simply grew his own.

A home garden is an easy and fun way to provide highly nourishing and often inexpensive foods for maximum health. During wars, many people grew their own fruits and vegetables on fire escapes. It doesn't take much space to grow a wide variety of foods.

Anyone can grow salad veggies, spices, and other incredibly tasty edibles, as well as medicinally useful plants for teas, whether they reside in Manhattan, Chicago, or Nome, Alaska. It's inexpensive, and when you grow it yourself you know for sure you're not eating pesticides.

DID YOU KNOW:

- Fifteen percent of Americans use organic growing methods in their gardens.
- A 100-square-foot garden can produce 10,000 servings of produce per year.[1]
- Many plants can be grown in pots on balconies or windowsills, even in the kitchen.
- You can grow your own cosmetically useful plants: aloe vera for burns; chamomile as a lightening hair rinse; lavender and sage as rinses for darker hair (see Chapter 42).
- Other herbs are excellent for protection against environmental pollution or as home remedies and can be consumed raw in salads, or used as teas. Alfalfa sprouted from seeds helps reduce cholesterol, has shown some evidence of cancer prevention, and "is one of the most nutritious foods known."[2] Your garden should never replace a trusted family doctor, but there is increasing and fascinating evidence supporting the potential medicinal benefits from foods you can grow in your own backyard. Yarrow, which has delicate bright flowers and loves the sun, fights fever.[3] Peppermint helps in the vomiting of pregnancy and the treatment of colds.[4] Garlic fights cancer, as well as reducing blood cholesterol.[5] Lavender, often used as a fragrance, soothes the nerves and stimulates sleep.[6] Rosemary strengthens the heartbeat.[7] Fennel can help with menstruation and menopause.[8]
- Although some people call dandelions "weeds," they are treasured by herbalists. The young leaves are nutritional powerhouses, chock full of vitamins and minerals, and make great salad fixings. In England, its root has been used to treat hepatitis.[9] (The root can also be used to make tea.[10]) Dill can help with colic and has been called "the herb of choice in the colic of children."[11]

SIMPLE THINGS TO DO

- Start with easy-to-grow greens and herbs for salads: Chinese garlic, chives, cilantro, dandelion, lettuce, oregano, sage, tarragon, and thyme.
- Even if you have a lot of shade you can grow leafy shoot vegetables such as lettuce and spinach that require only six hours of sunlight a day to keep salad bowls filled.[12] Others include arugula, cabbage, kale, and collards.
- Grow beets and turnip greens for both their above-ground shoots and below-ground roots. Also consider summer squash, cauliflower, broccoli, and asparagus.
- Containerize vegetables, if necessary, in large movable planters with casters or wheels. They can be moved to catch the sun as it changes during the growing season.
- Avoid growing edible plants near streets. No one wants to eat vehicle exhaust.

RESOURCES

Johnny's Selected Seeds
Foss Hill Road
Albion ME 04910-9731
(207)437-4301
Fax: (207)437-2165

Organic seeds, flowers, vegetables, herbs, and gardening supplies.

Natural Health magazine
P.O. Box 57320
Boulder CO 80322-7320

Information on herbal medicine, available at newsstands.

Organic Gardening magazine
P.O. Box 7320
Red Oak IA 51591

Information on growing fruits, vegetables, and herbs organically, available at newsstands.

30. Feminizing Jake

"Take a grape. Spray it with up to eighteen different pesticides, including DDT. Grow it in chemical fertilizer. Spray it some more with fungicide. Shrink wrap it and PRESTO, you have a raisin."

—Cesar Chavez

Call him Jake. He is a healthy American male. Perhaps he hangs out at the local fitness center pumping iron. Perhaps he bicycles daily along the seashore or the lake. He probably exercises three to four times a week. He is certainly interested in maintaining lifelong sexual potency and virility. So when it comes to his health, he wants to do everything right. He shops in gourmet markets, purchasing only the leanest, most expensive cuts of choice beef; he eats plenty of fresh fruits and vegetables. When he snacks, he prefers a healthy, natural sweet, like raisins, and when he has the son he's always wanted he'll make sure that his little boy eats plenty of raisins, too.

It all seems so right. But it isn't: Jake is dosing himself daily with environmental toxins; yet, he hasn't a clue. The results may well be catastrophic, both for his health—and that of his children.

In fact, it is men's exposure on a daily basis—and the exposure of their children—to a sea of pesticides and industrial pollutants that mimic the feminizing hormones known as estrogens, that may well underlie some of the most disturbing trends affecting male reproductive health.[1] These chemicals are suspected of faking out the body, crosscircuiting hormone systems and the development of male characteristics that should already be clearly forming in the unborn baby. Environmental chemicals which mimic estrogen in the body are called "xenoestrogens" (from the Greek word *xenos*, meaning foreign). Human studies are needed to determine whether increased chemical exposures are threatening the very basis of male sexuality.

DID YOU KNOW:

- It is suspected that increases in male diseases "may be related to exposure to pesticides and other . . . chemicals that can mimic [estrogens]."[2]
- Increasing incidence of testicular cancer and abnormalities, prostate cancer, and falling sperm counts are associated with exposure to chemicals that mimic hormones.[3,4,5,6,7,8,9,10,11]
- The prevalence of testicular cancer in Denmark has increased three to four times from the 1940s to the 1980s. Incidence is also increasing in Finland, Scotland, and the United States.[12]
- *You're only half the man your grandfather was.* A systematic review of sixty-one tests on semen quality involving some fifteen thousand men without a history of infertility revealed a fifty-percent reduction in average sperm count.
- Pregnant rats exposed to only one hundred parts per million per day of a commonly used fungicide gave birth to half-male, half-female offspring. These hermaphrodites (possessing both male and female sex organs) were incapable of reproducing. The pesticide, brand name Vinclozolin, is found in the food supply, particularly in wine.

SIMPLE THINGS TO DO

- Eat organic food (see Chapter 24).
- The most protective diet is whole grains, fresh fruits and vegetables, and olive oil with ocean fish (see Chapters 25 and 32).
- *I only wanted a Big Mac, not a sex change.* Quit chowing down on fast food burgers. They're loaded with female hormones that are prevalent in cattle. Purchase only naturally or organically

grown beef. (Make sure the label says the animals were raised without hormones; see Chapter 24.)

- Avoid plastic food packaging and canned foods whenever possible. Packaged and canned foods can be contaminated with carcinogenic and estrogenic contaminants that leach into the food from the packaging or lining.[13,14] Choose unwrapped and fresh foods when possible. Store freezer foods in plain, unbleached paper wrap.

31. You've Come a Long Way, Baby
. . . or Have You?

The environment has a profound influence on women's health concerns. Only recently has the scientific world begun to acknowledge the havoc that results in women's bodies from their exposure to environmental chemicals that mimic estrogens and interfere with their hormonal processes. Pesticides, certain plastics, and dioxins commonly found in red meat and dairy are leading suspects.

Did You Know:

- Endometriosis, a chronic pelvic disorder producing pain, heavy menstrual bleeding, and possibly infertility, affects five million women in the United States. One culprit appears to be exposure to environmental pollutants.[1] Eighty percent of monkeys exposed daily to dioxin, at low levels, developed endometriosis. The severity of the disease increased with the dose. Most women have traces of dioxin in their blood.[2] "It's highly improbable . . . that humans won't be responsive to dioxin."[3]
- Ovarian cancer is clearly related to environmental factors, including exposure to the weed-killing pesticide atrazine[4,5]
- Substantial evidence has been accumulating since the 1970s that breast cancer is related to environmental influences, particularly dietary toxins that the body mistakes for estrogens.[6,7,8,9,10]
- Dairy products have a possible special role as a risk factor for

breast cancer, possibly because of dietary contaminants, viruses, or naturally occurring hormones.[11,12,13,14,15,16]

- Some of the lowest rates of breast cancer are found among Japanese women who consume traditional Asian diets which are low in fats and made up of fruits, vegetables, grains, and fish. One feature of the Japanese diet is consumption of soybeans and foods made from them. In fact, the average Japanese citizen eats more than fifty pounds of soy-rich tofu every year. Such foods appear to be protective against breast cancer.[17,18,19]
- Soy foods are available in health food stores, gourmet markets, and many supermarkets. Soy milk, soy cheese, and tofu everything from hot dogs to dressing all have a positive impact on your health, including lowering cholesterol.
- Low rates of breast cancer are also found among women who consume high amounts of olive oil in their diet.
- Vegetables, including broccoli, brussels sprouts, cabbage, cauliflower, kale, mustard greens, and turnips, offer dietary protection against female cancer.[20]
- Cans and plastic containers can leach estrogen-mimicking substances into your food.[21]

SIMPLE THINGS TO DO

- Significantly reduce consumption of red meats. If you must, buy lean organic meats raised without pesticides or hormones. (See Chapter 24, Resources section.)
- Avoid plastic wraps on food or cooking in plastic containers. Glass is safest for cooking.
- Try to buy as many fresh foods as possible, avoiding canned foods and plastic containers.
- Limit your intake of dairy products.
- Eat soy foods as part of a balanced diet, unless you suffer from soy sensitivity.
- If your macho man doesn't think soy is "guy food," let him know it protects against heart disease. Pretty soon he'll be saying, "Honey, pass the tofu."
- Eat plenty of whole grains, fruits, and vegetables.

RESOURCES

National Women's Health Network

514 10th Street N.W., Suite 400
Washington DC 20004
(202)347-1140

Booklets on women and environmental health issues.

32. WHAT'S IN THE FRIDGE?

BACKGROUND

So you've read this far and you think the only things you can eat are tofu burgers and alfalfa sprouts. The thought of swearing off hot dogs, chips, burgers, fries, cheese, pizza, T-bones, doughnuts, diet sodas, and candy has you terrified. You're thinking of burning this book before anyone finds it and you go into Häagen-Dazs withdrawals. Your mind is racing . . . we will all die eventually anyway . . . have been eating stuff for years and am still alive . . . these guys must have stock in a root and tuber farm.

Chill out!

No one is perfect.

Absolutes are for God and IRS auditors.

You have some facts. That is a start. If you are making ten wrong food choices a day, maybe now you can cut it to six. If you gotta have it, have it. But here are some hints to help make a healthy diet easier and delicious.

SIMPLE THINGS TO DO

You don't have a garden. There are no health food stores around. And you don't have the money to shop for organic food. Now what?

OK to Eat

Turkey
Turkey, chicken hot dogs (no nitrite)
Turkey sausage and bacon (no nitrite)
Skinless chicken
Lean red meat (if any)
Deep-sea fish (see Chapter 25)
Pasta
Vegetables
Soy cheese
Balsamic rice
Fresh fruit juices
Fresh French and Italian breads without preservatives
Whole grain bread
Soda sweetened with fruit juice
Bananas, watermelon, cantaloupes
Brown sugar
Free range eggs
Low-fat or nonfat dairy products
Nonfat yogurt
Low-fat or nonfat frozen yogurt
Pizza bread, tomato sauce, and low-fat cheese (make your own pizza)
Baked chips
Pretzels
Herb teas
Honey
Olive oil

Not OK to Eat

Soda with caffeine or artificial sweetener
Popsicles, ice cream, Jell-O with artificial sweetener
Boxed cereals containing sugar, artificial colors, or preservatives
Pork bacon and sausage
Red meat with lots of fat and marbling
Fried chips
Fried foods
Margarine
Refined cooking oils
Artificial sweeteners (such as Nutrasweet and Sweet 'n Low)
Pork and beef hot dogs (with nitrite)
Soups and salad dressings with MSG

When You Can Have It All—Always Choose Organic

All of the following are available as organic foods:
Fruits and vegetables
Milk, cheeses, and butter
Meat
Pasta
Fruit juice
Grains, flours, and cereals
Vegetable oils
Eggs from veggie fed and free range chickens
Maple syrup
Coffee

When You've Got the Munchies—Go Organic!

The following are available in organic forms:
Organic licorice sweetened with molasses
Sherbet (fruit juice sweetened)
Crackers made from organic flour
Cookies made with organic flour and fruit juice sweetened
Juice popsicles
Popcorn

Pretzels
Ice cream and frozen yogurt
Granola bars
Peanuts, walnuts, pecans
Become a dual market shopper. Purchase what you can at your regular supermarket and try to shop at health food markets for organic foods and products.

RESOURCES

See Chapter 24.

Part IV

SHOP SMART

---- ✤ ----

33. I HAVE ONE WORD FOR YOU—PLASTIC

"Styrene is found in one hundred percent of human tissues. Opportunities for exposure to styrene abound. It may be present in drinking water, food, ambient air, exhaled cigarette smoke, in the workplace, or in consumer products, such as polystyrene-based disposal cups."

—FOUNDATION FOR ADVANCEMENTS
IN SCIENCE AND EDUCATION[1]

It's hard being a disco girl in the 90s. Sally's one consolation for working at Jimmy's Second Hand Music Store is getting all her Donna Summer disco CDs at half price. It's tough working the shrink-wrap machine, standing all day in white, patent leather disco boots, trying to make scuzzy, used CDs look like they're worth Jimmy's outrageous prices. At least, she doesn't have to worry about sitting down in her vinyl miniskirt while Joe the Lech drools across the floor. Sally's three-inch acrylic nails snag in the machine all day.

At lunchtime she grabs her pink plastic Barbie lunchbox and makes a beeline to her car—a pink '69 Corvette. It's a really nice car. Sally protects the leather with see-through seat covers. They're a little hot as she plops down. Ouch! But she jams in her Donna Summer CD and it wails on her eight-speaker stereo. Life is good. It's down to the "drive-thru" for her coffee and then to the park where she can eat in peace and dream of line-dancing with the Bee Gees. She hates these coffee cups, though. The stuff just sweats through the sides and drips all over the place. She hates the sandwich bags more—they're a bitch to open with three-inch nails. She squirts down a soft drink from her 7-11 souvenir sports bottle, and checks her watch. It's almost time for her doctor's appointment. You have to stay in shape if you want to be a disco girl!

When she arrives, her doctor looks concerned. "Sally, your cholesterol's perfect, but your blood is half plastic!"

"Oh," she says, unbothered. She's got something more important on her mind, rubbing her arm, then her leg. "Doctor, is this really my skin?"

Styrene is a plastic chemical found in literally every American. That's right—in you and me! Styrene is associated with a range of disorders including cancer, nerve damage, fatigue, and loss of memory.[2,3,4,5,6,7,8,9,10,11] How'd it get there? How about those fast-food cups and containers?

Plastic provides enormous benefits and makes life easier. Ask an athlete wearing protective headgear, a heart valve patient, or anybody leaving Blockbuster on a Friday night, arms filled with videos and CDs. But we don't need plastic everything.

DID YOU KNOW:

- NASA banned the use of polyvinyl chloride in space capsules because of toxic fumes.
- Recycle plastics, sure! But that's not the health problem. Manufacturing plastics is one of the largest sources of toxic wastes. They pollute our air, water, land—and us!
- Other plastics used in food packaging leach cancer-causing chemicals into food and beverages.[12,13]

SIMPLE THINGS TO DO

- Don't eat or drink out of polystyrene ("Styrofoam") containers.
- Buy fresh foods. Avoid plastic food packaging when you can.
- Tell store clerks you don't need a bag when you don't.
- Tell the dry cleaner to "hold" on the plastic wrap. It traps the dry-cleaning chemicals on your clothes, and those chemicals then concentrate in your closet. Or use the protective wrap until you get home and remove it and let your clothes air out on the porch, balcony, or in the garage before putting them away.

PAPER OR PLASTIC? . . . OR WHAT?

Products	Try These on for Size
Plastic shopping bags	Reusable canvas tote bags
Plastic sandwich bags	Waxed paper
Disposable diapers	Cloth diapers
Plastic-wrapped produce	Brown paper bags
Synthetic fiber carpets	Wool or cotton rugs
Synthetic fill mattresses	Cotton or down
Synthetic fill pillows	Cotton or down
Hot/cold beverage cups	Your own mug
PVC pipes	Copper pipes
Shower curtains	Glass doors
Floor tiles	Ceramic tiles
Soft drink bottles	Glass

RESOURCES

Plastic Alternatives

Co-Op America

2100 M St. N.W., Suite 310
Washington DC 20036
(202)872-5307

Earth Care Paper Co
100 S. Baldwin
Madison WI 53703
(608)256-5522

Real Recycled Catalog
1541 Adrian Road
Burlingame CA 94010
(800)233-5335

Activist Groups

Citizen's Clearinghouse for Hazardous Wastes
P.O. Box 6806
Falls Church VA 22040
(703)237-2249

The Entanglement Network c/o Defenders of Wildlife
1244 19th St. N.W.
Washington DC 20036
~~(202)659-9510~~

34. WAX YOUR CAR, NOT YOUR TUMMY

How would you like finding out that those shiny fruits and vegetables you're eating are coated in shellac?

The apples, cucumbers, watermelons, oranges, and beans glisten
in their supermarket bins. Nancy grabs a shiny cucumber. It slips
right out of her hand. Again she grabs it and again it rockets from
her hand. Johnny comes by and plucks an apple he can see himself
in. As he chomps down, the rest of the apples topple to the floor.

A store clerk starts frantically picking them up, but he's slipping and falling all over the place. In fact, everybody nearby starts slipping, sliding, and falling down. The aisle has been transformed into a skating rink! Someone glides by doing a *moon walk*. "Hey, who waxed the floors?" shouts Johnny.

Many of the fruits and vegetables you purchase at the supermarket are coated with wax. Those sparkling apples and cucumbers weren't grown that way. Most consumers don't realize they are eating waxes made from shellac and petrochemicals, such as polyethylene, with their food.[1] Waxes have no nutritional value. They are only used for cosmetics and to extend shelf life.

DID YOU KNOW:

- Chemical fungicides are added to wax to prevent mold.[2]
- Federal law requires retailers to have a posted sign stating if bulk produce has been waxed.[3] Have you seen any signs lately? After all, would you rather buy an apple with, or without, shellac?
- Penalties for not posting notice signs include fines up to one thousand dollars and one year in jail. Seen any grocers in jail lately?
- Fruits and vegetables that are commonly waxed include apples, watermelons, squash, oranges, potatoes, tomatoes, nuts, tangerines, avocados, peppers, eggplants, papayas, onions, coconuts, and pineapples.
- Rinsing fruits and vegetables with water only does not remove wax or pesticides.
- Many local farmers' markets don't wax or spray fungicides on foods because they are sold quickly.

THEY DON'T EVEN PUT THESE IN CAR WAX	
Fungicide	Health Hazard
Benomyl	Cancer. Birth defects.[4,5]
Dicloran and Imazalil	Poorly tested.[6]
Ortho-phenylphenol	Cancer. Suppresses immune system.[7]
Sodium ortho-phenyl phenate	Cancer.[8]

SIMPLE THINGS TO DO

- Buy organic fruits and vegetables (see Chapter 24).
- Shop at farmers' markets.
- Hot water and soap will remove most of the wax from fruits and vegetables. But remember, some pesticides are in the edible portions of the food itself.

Go Straight to Jail, Don't Pass Go, Don't Collect $200

Write a letter. Demand that your local supermarket comply with the labeling law: Food and Drug Administration Compliance Policy Guides; Chapter 20—Food General; Guide 7120.08: Safety and Labeling of Waxed Fruits and Vegetables. Quote them chapter and verse, and if the store won't do anything, report it to:

Director Division of Regulatory Guidance
Center for Food Safety and Applied Nutrition
Department of Health and Human Services
Food and Drug Administration
200 C St. S.W.
Washington DC 20204

Copy your local state health department, and newspapers.

RESOURCES

Americans for Safe Foods

Center for Science and the Public Interest
1501 16th St. N.W.
Washington DC 20036
(202)332-9110

Information on waxed produce.

Citizen Petition

34 Nathan Lord Road
Amherst NH 03031
(603)673-7849

Provides information on waxed fruit and vegetable issues.

35. SNOW WHITE HAS A BLACK HEART

"Chlorine bleaching of wood pulp leaves a toxic legacy in much of the paper we encounter: coffee filters, disposable diapers, paper towels, milk cartons, newspapers, and facial tissues."

—JANET RALOFF[1]

A pure white backdrop. White towels. White wicker chair. White rug. A woman is in a seamless, sheer white dress. Narrow arms and hands fitted seductively in white gloves that stretch beyond the elbow. Nothing moves. Different shapes, barely distinguishable, are camouflaged in white. The pale flesh tones of her face define the scene, as they scintillate and resonate with the music. Her vamp lipstick blushes the only color in the landscape. A new Madonna video? Well, almost: it's a bleach commercial.

Americans have been conditioned to associate white with antiseptic and virginal cleanliness. That's why we have Snow White and Madonna. Well, Snow White.

Ironically, bleached white underwear, tampons, paper, napkins, milk cartons, toilet paper, egg cartons, paper towels, and coffee filters all contain traces of dioxin, which is highly toxic.[2,3,4,5,6,7] Tests find this potent toxin in the tissues of virtually every American.[8,9] The EPA reports that levels in the population are high enough to cause infertility, immune system damage, and cancer.[10,11,12,13,14,15,16]

Did You Know:

- When chlorine combines with heat and certain materials, dioxins are formed. Wood pulp is chlorine-bleached to make white paper products. The waste, containing dioxins, is discharged into rivers and streams.
- A minnow accumulates in its tissues one hundred sixty thousand times the level of dioxin present in the water and sediment around it.[17]
- We become contaminated by both the paper products and the fish.[18]
- A single ounce of dioxin could kill one million people.[19]
- Dioxin has been shown to leach from cartons into milk.
- Dioxin leaches from paper trays into microwaved foods.
- Forty to seventy percent of the dioxin in bleached coffee filters can leach into your coffee.
- Waste incinerators release dioxin into the air.
- The average American receives one hundred sixty-six times the dioxin dose recommended by an EPA science advisory board.[20]
- Each year, *Time* magazine uses approximately forty-five thousand tons of bleached paper, leading to the discharge of more than one hundred fifty thousand pounds of bleached wastes into our waters.[21]

Simple Things to Do

- Use unbleached coffee filters.
- Buy milk in glass bottles.
- Avoid fish caught from waters near pulp and paper mills.
- Buy nonbleached paper products for home and office.
- Don't microwave food in paper packaging. Use microwave-safe glass.
- Substitute nonchlorine alternatives for laundry, such as hydrogen peroxide.
- Call *Time* magazine at (800)843-TIME and demand they honor their pledge to use totally chlorine-free paper.

Resources

Nonbleach Paper Products

Atlantic Recycled Paper Company
(800)323-2811

Cross Pointe Paper Corporation
(800)543-3297

Earth Care
(800)347-0070

Lyn-Bar
(800)729-3117

Real Recycled
(800)233-5335

Seventh Generation
(800)456-1177

Educational Materials

Greenpeace Public Information Booklets
1436 U St. N.W.
Washington DC 20009
(202)319-2444
Internet address: http://www.greenpeace.org/

36. There Goes the Ozone

"What does it mean to redefine one's relationship to the sky? What will it do to our children's outlook on life if we have to teach them to be afraid to look up?"

—Vice President Al Gore[1]

You grab sunblock number one hundred ninety-eight, three pairs of sunglasses, three umbrellas, and two hats that cover your ears. You put on a long-sleeved shirt, pants, socks, and sandals. You get to the beach and sit there, buried under your clothing, sweating and suffocating. You feel like a caveman. You don't know why you are wearing all this stuff . . . a friend told you . . . who heard it on TV . . . something about skin cancer and premature wrinkling. All you know is it is no fun going to the beach anymore.

You've also heard something about the ozone. Indeed, if it weren't for what remains of the ozone layer in the sky, we'd all be fried dumplings by now.[2] The problem is that industrial pollutants in the sky have been breaking down ozone. Since 1985, scientists have been documenting this gap in the ozone—the ozone "hole"— which is spreading from Antarctica to heavily populated areas. Due to this spreading hole, more of the sun's harmful ultraviolet (UV) radiation is leaking into the earth's atmosphere.

The hot news is that the ozone is about as thin as parchment paper and growing thinner with every passing year, and that this depletion is now occurring in the spring and summer, the time of the year when the sun's rays are the most direct and able to do the most damage. That means that we have a serious health problem—too much sun is getting through.

DID YOU KNOW:

- If ozone loss reaches ten percent by the year 2000, as expected, there will be about a quarter of a million additional cases of skin cancer annually in the United States, and an estimated four thousand more deaths.
- Excess UV exposure is thought to cause cataracts. More than a million additional cases of cataracts will occur by the end of this decade because of increasing UV exposure.
- There is evidence that ozone depletion is damaging people's immune systems, harming their ability to fight infectious disease.[3] This happens before they lose protection against sunburn.[4] How dark the skin is doesn't seem to matter.[5]
- One in six Americans will develop skin cancer in their lifetime.[6] The incidence of a deadly skin cancer form of melanoma is pres-

ently rising at a faster rate than that of any other cancer. In 1935, the risk of developing melanoma in the United States during one's lifetime was one in fifteen hundred. Today it's one in one hundred five.

- Sunbathers should not be overly confident with sunscreen. It may not protect against the growth of skin cancer that began in childhood.[7]

SIMPLE THINGS TO DO

- During the summer, use a sunscreen with a sun protection factor of twenty-five to thirty. Sunscreens over thirty are irritating. Apply liberally fifteen to thirty minutes *before* exposure to allow it to penetrate and still leave a protective layer on the skin's surface. Remember, even a twenty-minute exposure when you're running errands at lunch takes its toll on your skin over time. Use sunscreen.
- Don't bake in the sun.
- Stay out of the sun during peak hours between ten to two (or eleven to three during Daylight Savings Time).
- Use a beach umbrella.
- If you are around reflective surfaces, including sand, snow, concrete, and water, use protection.
- Don't be fooled when it is cool, wet, or cloudy. You can receive a hefty dose of radiation even on a cloudy, cool, or wet day.
- Apply sunscreen frequently while in the sun.
- Even if you are using a waterproof sunscreen, reapply it after you go in the water or after perspiring.
- Every adult should take one hundred micrograms of selenium daily during summer months, and individuals with a history of cancer of any kind should take two hundred micrograms daily.[8]

For children, follow these additional guidelines:

- It may not be possible to always keep your kids indoors during periods of peak exposure. Still, do your best. Put sunscreen on

before school if your kids will be playing outside at lunch or going on a field trip.
- The tender skin of babies and young children is especially vulnerable to burns. Keep very young infants off the beach, older babies covered up in the shade. Begin using sunscreen on children at six months.

Hey Bugs, Got Any Carrots on You?

The evidence that your diet is a critical aspect of cataract prevention is becoming stronger every year. Eating correctly and taking your vitamins and minerals—particularly beta-carotene (a form of vitamin A), vitamins C and E, and selenium—may have a big influence on your eyesight as you age, and as the ozone layer gets even thinner.

Take up to one gram of vitamin C three times daily together with up to eight hundred international units of vitamin E, two hundred thousand international units of beta-carotene, and up to two hundred micrograms of selenium.[9] Check with your doctor.

Avoid rancid foods and increase your consumption of yellow vegetables (rich in beta-carotene) and other vitamin-rich fresh fruits and vegetables. Such a diet, together with intelligent and early use of dietary supplements, is a prescription for vision for life.

As for sunglasses:

- Buy ones that specify how much UV radiation they block. Get one with the highest value. Don't count on sunglasses that have no UV protection rating.
- Wraparound sunglasses block out more UV radiation.

RESOURCES

Greenpeace
1436 U St. N.W.
Washington DC 20009
(202)462-1177
Fax: (202)462-4507

Order the reports The Effects of Ozone Destruction *for further information on the effects of ozone depletion and* Climbing out of the Ozone Hole, A Preliminary Survey of Alternatives to Ozone-Depleting Chemicals *for information on ozone-friendly technologies.*

37. VOTING AT THE CHECKOUT LINE

"For the first time in my forty-year lifetime, people are standing up in large numbers and saying a simple and vitally important thing: Being a good human being is good business."

—PAUL HAWKEN,
author of *The Ecology of Commerce*

Joe Blow goes to the polls every year and votes for the candidate with the flashiest smile and most hair mousse. Joe's sly: he once took out a classified that read, "Wanted: Winning Lottery Tickets (will pay 10% finder's fee)." The hippest commercial moves him. He drinks Gatorade like Mike. He wears Nikes like Andre. He eats Nutrasweet because Cher tells him to. He bought Windows 95 because he loves the Rolling Stones. Joe's hip. He's a Madison Avenue type guy. Joe buys stuff with the same intelligence that he uses to vote.

If we all voted in political elections the way Joe does, we would end up with the guy with the best media handlers as president instead of the best guy for the job. But we don't. We try to research the candidates and issues. We should also research the products we buy, but no matter how hard we try, most of us vote at the checkout line with the same information as Joe. Most household product labels don't tell us anything. All we've got is Madison Avenue hype.

If Joe Blow prefers his cleanser with crystalline silica, furniture polish with formaldehyde, window cleaner with butyl cellosolve, that's fine. It is a free market. If he wants his raisins with DDT, he can buy them to munch while he watches reruns of *Beavis and Butt-head*. But in a truly free market where labels tell all, most of us, who are concerned about our family's health, would choose other products. Manufacturers and food growers would respond by making products and foods and beverages safer.

DID YOU KNOW:

- Absolutely no regulations have ever been passed by Congress that require manufacturers to tell consumers all the ingredients in household products. That means when you pick up a can of Ajax powder you will never be told it contains crystalline silica, a fine dust associated with lung cancer in workers who do industrial sandblasting and polishing.[1,2] You will never know, from the label, that Olde English Lemon Furniture Polish (pump) contains formaldehyde, which also causes cancer and allergic reactions.[3] Or that Lysol spray contains the chemical disinfectant ortho-phenylphenol, and that the EPA classifies it as cancer causing.[4]

- If you call Procter & Gamble and other companies, their customer service representatives sometimes deny shoppers information on ingredients. (We know; we tried.)

- The California raisin growers currently use a pesticide that contains cancer-causing DDT. Residues of this freshly sprayed pesticide are found in school lunches.[5] Yet, no law requires the raisin growers to tell you.

- Under regulations of the Occupational Safety and Health Administration (OSHA), men and women who work in factories are entitled to information on toxic chemicals used on the job. Homemakers, however, are not considered "workers"—even though they handle the same chemicals as factory workers, and levels of contamination of some chemicals in homes can be hundreds of times greater than in factories. Homemakers are *not* legally entitled to information on the hazardous chemicals present in products that they use.

- Many scientists and consumers are justifiably concerned that BGH, a growth hormone used to synthetically increase cows' milk production, produces high levels of tumor-stimulating chemicals in your milk. Yet, the federal government generally prohibits producers of BGH-free milk from labeling their products as being free from this potent substance. However, some states have passed their own legislation permitting such labeling.

- Sales of organic foods skyrocketed in 1994 by twenty-two percent, the fifth straight year sales increased more than twenty percent, making this one of the nation's leading growth industries.[6] Interestingly, the bulk of this growth was not from health food stores, but from mainstream supermarkets, where sales increased from ninety-four million dollars in 1993 to nearly one hundred eighty-eight million in 1994. Consumer shopping habits are undergoing a major change throughout America. This is an indication of the power of information and the impact it can have on the market.

SIMPLE THINGS TO DO

- Form your own company to get the real information you need on what's in household products. If your name is Jane, call it **Jane Clean.** If your name is Harold, call it **Harry Clean.** You may even want to create some stationery just to make it all that more official.
- Once in business, you are legally entitled to receive the same information that factory workers receive. This information is contained in "material safety data sheets" (MSDSs) that provide information on hazardous ingredients in products, health effects, and safe handling procedures.
- Call the 800 number listed on the product you are purchasing, or write to the corporation, and tell the customer service representative that you represent **Jane Clean** or **Harry Clean** and that you need to obtain an MSDS for the products under OSHA regulations.
- Once you've obtained the information, you can see what's in the product you're using. If the ingredients are not to your liking, make the same requests for other products. You will find some are very safe.
- Support organized boycotts against foods or products substantiated as unsafe.
- Another excellent source for health information on toxins is The Community Right to Know provisions of the federal Compre-

hensive Environmental Response, Compensation and Liability Act of 1980 (CERCLA), which was set up to deal with the hazards from toxic waste dumps.

RESOURCES

The Safe Shopper's Bible (Macmillan 1995)

By David Steinman & Samuel S. Epstein, M.D. The key shopper's resource to brand-name household products, cosmetics, and foods.

Chemtrec

2501 M St. N.W.
Washington DC 20037
(800)262-8200
Fax: (202)463-1596

Chemtrec provides MSDSs to the general public for many types of products at no charge. (Many companies, however, refuse to release their MSDSs even through Chemtrec.)

CERCLA Hot Line

(800)424-9346

Excellent source for health information on toxins.

Green Seal

1730 Rhode Island Avenue N.W., Suite 1050
Washington DC 20036
(202)331-7337
(202)331-7333

Provides product endorsements for a wide variety of consumer goods which are healthy for you and the environment.

The National Green Pages

Co-op America
1612 K Street N.W., Suite 600
Washington DC 20006
(202)872-5307

A definitive, national listing of environmental services and products.

Part V

LOOKING GOOD

---

38. PUT A PRETTY FACE ON

"Contrary to what is popular belief, the Federal Food and Drug Administration does not test cosmetics for safety as it does food and drugs. The FDA does not have the authority to require that manufacturers prove the safety of products before their marketing. . . . Even if the agency suspects that serious adverse health effects are caused by a cosmetic product, the agency can't ask for ingredient information from the manufacturer to determine the formulation, or require that the manufacturer provide test data to prove the product safety or efficacy."

—CONGRESSMAN RON WYDEN[1]

Let's play a word-association game. We'll give you the words. You tell us what comes to mind first. The first word is makeup . . . you know, mascara . . . foundation . . .

If you came up with beauty, you might be surprised to know that hazardous waste might be more accurate.

A hazardous waste dump is probably the last thing you think of when putting on your makeup in the morning, or at night when you're dressed to the nines. Commercial brands of facial makeup are loaded with a wide range of UNDISCLOSED chemicals that can cause cancer, nerve and reproductive damage, and birth defects, as well as allergies and irritation—and that's only the beginning.

The funny thing is, it does not need to be that way. Indeed, many companies make cosmetic products that are great. They are pure. They are natural and safe.

DID YOU KNOW:

- Many commercial brands of cosmetics and personal care products contain the chemicals diethanolamine and triethanolamine, also abbreviated as DEA and TEA, and often shown on a label attached with other ingredients, as in "cocamide-DEA," or "TEA-sodium lauryl sulfate." Both DEA and TEA interact with other chemicals in products, while in stores or medicine cabinets, to form cancer-causing chemicals called nitrosamines.[2,3,4,5,6,7,8]
- The longer the chemicals in cosmetics remain on your skin, the more they can enter your body.
- Thirty-seven percent of the products tested by the FDA contained nitrosamines.[9]
- Nitrosamines in cigarette smoke cause cancer.[10] Tobacco is the leading source of nitrosamine exposure in the United States.[11] The next leading source . . . COSMETICS![12]
- Frequent use of facial makeup during pregnancy is associated with a sixty-percent increased risk for childhood brain tumors.[13]
- The German government isn't waiting. Their cosmetics are unlikely to contain nitrosamines, because the German Federal Health Office in 1987 discouraged manufacturers from using DEA and TEA.[14]
- Many of the preservatives used in cosmetics and personal care products contain or release formaldehyde, which causes cancer, nerve damage, allergies, and irritation, as well as acting as a sensitizer (the body becomes sensitive to that specific chemical and can then develop sensitivity to other chemicals).[15,16,17,18,19,20,21]

- Two formaldehyde-releasing cosmetic preservatives, imidazolidinyl urea and quaternium 15, are leading causes of skin problems in users.[22]
- Safer preservatives that do not contain or release formaldehyde include methylchoroisothiazolinone,[23] methylchloroisothiazolinone,[24] and parabens (butyl, ethyl, methyl, propyl).[25]
- The absolute most gentle preservatives include[26] grapefruit seed extract,[27] phenoxyethanol,[28] potassium sorbate,[29] sorbic acid,[30] vitamin E (tocopherol),[31] vitamin A (retinol),[32] and vitamin C (ascorbic acid).[33] Products containing these are the ones you should prefer whenever possible.
- A single commercial cosmetic or personal care product may contain any or all of these ingredients.

SIMPLE THINGS TO DO

- Read labels.
- Avoid products containing DEA or TEA!
- Choose products containing the safest preservatives (see the table below).

COMMON COSMETIC PRESERVATIVES

Least Safe	Safer	Safest
Bronopol	Methylchoroisothiazolinone	Grapefruit seed extract
Diazolidinyl urea	Methylisothiazolinone	Phenoxyethanol
DMDM hydantoin	Parabens (butyl, ethyl, methyl, propyl)	Potassium sorbate
Formaldehyde		Sorbic acid
Imidazolidinyl urea		Vitamin A (retinol)
Quaternium 15		Vitamin C (ascorbic acid)
		Vitamin E (tocopherol)

- Don't fall for brands just because they bill themselves as "natural." Many may contain a few plant extracts but are otherwise loaded with hidden and potentially hazardous ingredients.
- Shop at your local health food store. Look for brands from Aubrey Organics, Dr. Hauschka, Ecco Bella, Ida Grae, Logona, Mera, Paul Penders, and Weleda. Most of their products fulfill every criterion for being both natural and safe.

RESOURCES

The Safe Shopper's Bible (Macmillan 1995)

A complete brand-name guide to safe cosmetics and personal care products by David Steinman and Samuel S. Epstein, M.D.

39. I SMELL A RAT

"Low levels of the chemicals found in perfume can adversely affect the body in profound and subtle ways."

—IRENE WILKENFELD[1]

You've got a hot date, you're spicing up a marriage, or just skipping a shower. You splash on cologne, aftershave, or perfume. Now you're face to face with your date and you find out you must have a "drop-dead" bod, because your date just did!

DID YOU KNOW:

- Six hundred or more chemical ingredients may be used in a single scent.[2]
- Ninety-five percent of chemicals used in scents are derived from petroleum. "Many chemicals found in fragrances are designated as hazardous waste disposal chemicals."[3] They cause allergies

and irritation, as well as cancer, nerve damage, and birth defects.[4,5,6,7]

- Petroleum chemicals in perfumes cost less than ten dollars a pound. Natural ingredients such as jasmine cost more than ten thousand dollars a pound.[8] Which do you think you get?
- Symptoms reported by people sensitive to perfumes include spaciness, nausea, restlessness, irritability, anger, memory lapses, headaches, and sinus pain.[9]
- Fragrances are the leading cause of allergic reactions to cosmetics.[10]
- If you can smell a chemical, you are being exposed to the toxic chemicals from which it is made.[11]
- Though reported in 1984 to cause nerve damage, musk ambrette's production has increased six hundred percent.[12]
- Perfume in kitty litter and other fragranced products triggers asthma attacks.[13]
- "In the United States, supermarkets are about to start piping in the smell of freshly baked bread and other smells to attract the olfactory interest of the public."[14]

Venus Fly Trap

Could fragrance manufacturers possibly know that fragrance chemicals, some with narcotic properties, affect your nervous system? Seen any perfume commercials lately? How about this one from the fragrance industry . . .

"We will see fragrances pumped into factories where laborers are doing repetitive jobs. They will be used in nursing homes, hospitals, subways and prisons. . . ."[15]

SIMPLE THINGS TO DO

- Buy unscented or fragrance-free household products and cosmetics.
- If you must have a scent, purchase essential oils at your local

health food store, including rose, orange, lemon, and lavender. One drop goes a long, long way.
- Use baking soda to absorb room odors.
- Fresh flowers add a pleasant fragrance to rooms.

RESOURCES

Essential Oils

Aura Cacia

P.O. Box 3157
Santa Rosa CA 95402
(707)795-1312

Leydet Oils

P.O. Box 2354
Fair Oaks CA 95628
(916)965-7546

Oshadhi

R. J. F., Inc.
32422 Alipaz, Suite C
San Juan Capistrano 92675
(714)240-1104

Organizations

Citizens for a Toxic-Free Marin

400 Canal St., Suite 329
San Rafael CA 94901
(415)485-6870

Provides a highly informative, well-researched newsletter on the hazards of scents, perfumes, and fragrances.

Human Ecology Action League

P.O. Box 49126
Atlanta GA 30359
(404)248-1898

Supports individuals who are sensitive to chemicals. Publishes the comprehensive newsletter The Human Ecologist.

40. DON'T GET DIRTY IN THE SHOWER

"Contaminated water in the home can cause toxic exposures from cooking, dish and clothes washing, or during the flushing of toilets. Of singular importance is the use of . . . contaminated water for bathing and showering."

—JEFFREY LYBARGER, M.D.[1]

Janis Thompson, of Brentwood, California, was a power athlete. She ran. She played volleyball. She was in super shape.

She also ate plenty of fresh fruits, vegetables, and whole grains. She didn't smoke. She drank bottled water. So what the heck was happening? On a visit to her doctor, Janis admitted she was tired and suffering depression and mental fatigue, and often found herself in a drunkenlike stupor. Her physician, knowledgeable in environmental medicine, recognized the symptoms as potentially the result of solvent exposure. Having ordered a solvent screen (see Chapter 17), Janis learned that she had high levels of an industrial solvent, trichloroethylene (TCE), circulating in her blood. The TCE, a common drinking water contaminant, was damaging her nervous system, and the result was chronic fatigue accompanied by other symptoms. It could also cause cancer.

This couldn't be, Janis protested. She ate organic foods, exercised, and drank only bottled water. Where did this stuff come from? Due to her intense workouts, Janis showered three times a day. While she didn't drink the water, the shower's steam contained TCE that she breathed. She was becoming dirty in her own shower. She subsequently had her water tested, and it was loaded with TCE.

Did You Know:

- Many contaminants in tap water become gases at room temperature. Such substances are known in scientific lingo as volatile organic chemicals (VOCs).
- In fact, VOCs are absorbed and inhaled so efficiently, they are even more dangerous in the shower than in a single glass of tap water.[2,3]
- It has been observed that VOC contamination in water intended for uses other than drinking is a "substantial source of human exposure."[4] In fact, one's exposure from air is "substantially greater than that from water ingestion . . ."[5]
- Other "hidden" sources of exposure to VOCs include washing dishes, flushing toilets, boiling water, washing your face, and bathing.
- Many VOCs are skin and eye irritants. Elimination of such contaminants in shower and bath water can help clear up eyes and skin.

Simple Things to Do

- Install a shower filter. It will cost about fifty dollars. The work can be done by a plumber for a nominal fee.

Not So Simple Thing to Do

- If your water is really polluted or if you are particularly sensitive to chemicals, you might want to consider a whole-house water filter. This could cost $1500 to $2000, but it will filter all the water used in your home.

Resources

Nigra Enterprises
5699 Kanan Road
Agoura CA 91301
(818)889-6877

Stocks several types of shower filters.

41. A Smile That Won't Kill You

"Faye Dores was only thirty-five when in 1985 she was told that the severity of her ailments, including arthritis, colitis, fatigue, and memory loss, was so great that she would spend the rest of her life confined to a wheelchair. By late August of that year, all of her mercury fillings had been removed from her mouth. Within three weeks of their removal, she no longer required a cane and the rest of her symptoms began to disappear."

—"Is There Poison in Your Mouth?"
CBS News *60 Minutes*[1]

Who would have ever thought "a smile that kills" could literally do just that? In fact, one of the body's most hazardous toxic sites could be your mouth. Some two hundred thirty-five million Americans have mercury-based fillings. Known also as "silver" fillings or mercury "amalgams," most fillings are currently made from mercury combined with other metal. It is the mercury, making up about half the mix and added as a hardener, that is of critical importance to your health.[2] It causes brain damage and birth defects. It may be a cause of other diseases, and it's being put in people's mouths every time they have a filling!

In the United States, the official position of the dental community has been that the mercury in fillings is stable when mixed with other metals.[3] This concoction is safe, said the American Dental Association (ADA) in a March 30, 1995, position statement.

However, "now a growing number of scientists, doctors and dentists are saying mercury amalgams should be banned."[4] Some countries consider mercury fillings dangerous both to those who have them in their mouths and those who put them in your teeth. Germany and Sweden have banned the use of mercury as dental filling material.

DID YOU KNOW:

- In Northern Europe, the term for mercury was "quaksilber"—a forerunner of our English term "quicksilver." A dentist who used mercury was called a "quaksilber placer," or "quak" for short. Hence, the original use of the word "quack" was taken from dentists who used mercury for fillings.[5]
- In 1986, the ADA changed its code of ethics, making it a violation for any dentist to recommend the removal of amalgam because of mercury.[6] Who are the "quacks" now?
- Chewing and corrosion release tiny particles of mercury. This mercury gas travels to the brain and other areas of the body. Mercury particles also enter the lungs where they are transported into the bloodstream.[7]
- The amount of mercury detected in a person's mouth after chewing for ten minutes is ninety-two times higher than the mercury-vapor level in a newly painted room and three times higher than the United States government allows in the workplace.[8]
- The level of mercury in the breath after chewing is more than fifteen times greater in people with silver-amalgam fillings than those who do not have them.
- The two most dangerous sources of mercury for most people are diet, particularly seafood, and mercury amalgam fillings.[9]
- Mercury damages the nervous system. In the old days in England, hatters hand-rubbed mercury into felt to make it stiff enough to stand up for those big hats that were the rage. Their

bodies absorbed it through their skin. They got the shakes and became mentally "unstable." That is how the expression "mad as a hatter" came into being.[10]

- Parkinson's disease has been strongly related to high body levels of mercury.[11]

- A small 1990 study provides evidence that Alzheimer's patients have significantly higher than normal levels of mercury. The brains from ten autopsied Alzheimer's patients were compared with twelve brains of those whose deaths were from other causes. The investigators concluded that, "elevation of mercury in brains [of those with Alzheimer's] is the most important of the imbalances we observed. . . . This and our previous studies suggest that mercury toxicity plays a role in Alzheimer's disease."[12] While this does not prove a relationship between mercury and Alzheimer's disease, it points out again how people are exposed to dangerous chemicals before all the potential health effects are known.

- In a case reported in 1982, a seventeen-year-old girl went from "good grades, lots of friends, a cheerleader" to somebody "who dropped out of school . . . had become introverted . . . [with] severe pains in the chest, a reversion to childlike speaking, and a concern about dying." Her dentist traced the onset of attacks to about the same time she had mercury amalgam fillings put in her mouth. Once the amalgams were removed, "the attacks stopped."[13]

- In a study of twenty-two patients suffering severe chemical sensitivities, including allergies and chronic infections, "removal of dental mercury ('amalgam') fillings was the single most effective method of improving the health of these patients."[14]

- Patients have been shown to have "marked improvement" in immune system function after the removal of their mercury fillings.[15]

- Symptoms of mercury toxicity mimic a wide range of other conditions, especially arthritis, alcohol intoxication, immune system dysfunction, and stomach disturbances. Additional symptoms include depression, fearfulness, frequent bouts of anger, hallucinations, inability to accept criticism and to concentrate, indecision, irritability, memory loss, metallic taste, persecution complex, tremors of hands, head, lips, tongue, jaw, or eyelid, and weight loss.

- Signs of mercury in the mouth can take the form of dental disease and include receding, bleeding, or ulcerated gums; bone loss; foul breath; lesions; raised thickened white patches; inflammation; a burning sensation inside the cheeks or in the throat; tissue pigmentation; and blue marks at the gum line near to the mercury-amalgam filling.

SIMPLE THINGS TO DO

- If you suspect mercury poisoning, your doctor can order a mercury urine test.
- If you or a family member has to have a tooth filled, examine with your dentist safer alternatives to mercury fillings.
- Just because a filling has no mercury does not mean that your body will be compatible with it. Be careful before having mercury fillings removed. Since many alternative fillings contain other toxic ingredients, replacement of one toxic filling with another is unhealthy, unwise, and could be a waste of money. Insist on a material compatibility test to see if alternative materials are safe for you.
- Keep in mind that electrical readings on fillings may also be crucial. Electrical readings are taken for the purpose of identifying the sequence for removing fillings.[16]
- Use dentists who are well trained in all safety procedures.

RESOURCES

Environmental Dental Association
(619)586-1208

Foundation for Toxic Free Dentistry
Box #608010
Orlando FL 32860

Huggins Diagnostic Center
5080 List Drive, at Centennial
Colorado Springs CO 80919
(800)331-2303

Patient Support Group
Dental Amalgam Mercury Syndrome
Box #19032
Denver CO 80219

Serum Compatibility Test
(800)331-2303

42. HAIR DYES TO DIE FOR

"No matter how hazardous the chemicals used in hair dyes may be, the FDA has no power to ban them."

—Consumer Reports[1]

Detective Jake Moran was stymied. There were no clues, except a broken bottle of black hair dye in the bathroom sink and the body. The victim, Nancy Doe, seemed like an ordinary woman. Her neighbors said she came and went in all ways predictable. A friend, Lisa, told Jake that Nancy secretly craved wild and passionate sex with Wayne Newton but was always too inhibited to do anything about it. Her diary revealed a penchant for violence: she wanted to break both of Newt Gingrich's legs, but that was something she had in common with a lot of women her age. No, there was no sex, drugs, or violence in her untimely and premature death. Then the coroner's report came: Nancy Doe died of non-Hodgkin's lymphoma, one of the most common cancers which is also associated with long-term use of hair dyes. Holding the product label in his hand, Jake went to bust his suspect, except there was no law against death by hair dyes.

Maybe only Nancy and her hairdresser knew for sure. But what they didn't know, what no one told them, was that hair dyes cause cancer. The tragedy is that fifty million women and ten percent of men between thirty-five and sixty, in the United States, use hair dyes.[2] The trouble is that, in spite of substantial incriminating evidence, the people in the cosmetic industry don't want men and women to know their dirty little secret, and the law protects them from having to divulge the facts to the public.[3] Is this a conspiracy between FDA, Congress, and the hair dye manufacturers to get away with murder? Where's Oliver Stone when we need him?

Hair dyes cause cancer. If you're using them, you're at risk. You don't need them. You have safer alternatives.

DID YOU KNOW:

- Users and applicators of permanent and semipermanent hair dyes are at increased risk of non-Hodgkin's lymphoma, bone cancer, and Hodgkin's disease.[4,5,6,7,8,9,10,11,12]
- National Cancer Institute researchers estimate that the use of permanent and semipermanent hair dyes could account for as much as twenty percent of all cases of non-Hodgkin's lymphoma among United States women.[13]
- Men's products contain lead acetate, which causes cancer and enhances the toxic effects of other chemicals.[14,15] Lead acetate is absorbed through the skin.
- Other men's brands contain the same cancer-causing dyes used in women's products.
- Hair dyes are also a risk to children whose mothers used them just before conception or during pregnancy. The risk of childhood cancer could be increased by as much as ten times.[16,17,18]
- In spite of substantial evidence, a loophole in the 1938 Federal Food, Drug and Cosmetic Act exempts popular brands of hair dyes from desperately needed label warnings.[19]

SIMPLE THINGS TO DO

- Avoid using any product with the word "phenylenediamine" on the ingredients label. This is the stuff that can cause cancer.

- If you insist on using such dyes, delay their use as long as possible. The age women start using hair dyes can determine risk. Women who start at forty have a one-third less risk than those who start at thirty, while women who start at age twenty have an even higher risk.[20]
- Use the lightest shades. Most of the cancer risk is from darker shades. Women who use black, brown/brunette, and red hair dyes have higher risks than women who use lighter color dyes.[21]
- Use coloring methods that reduce the contact between the dye and your scalp. These include frosting and highlighting techniques such as tipping, streaking, or painting.
- If you insist on using commercial dyes, the safest are temporary dyes and rinses.
- Bleaches are safer than colorants.
- Hair colorings using pure henna, chamomile, or other herbs are much safer than commercial hair coloring products. Light Mountain Henna Gray claims to entirely cover gray when its two-step process is used according to instructions.
- One highly recommended line of natural colorants is Igora Botanic, available at salons. Their plant-based, semipermanent hair colors are composed exclusively of raw materials found in nature such as indigo, chamomile, and walnut that are able to produce subtle variations.
- An option for women who desire to entirely cover their gray is a permanent hair coloring product from VitaWave of California (see the Resources list).
- *You can make your own homemade rinses to bring out both highlights and color.* Experiment with different amounts of the ingredients mentioned below in order to perfect a blend that works best for your own hair color.
- The following rinses work best for blondes and naturally fair-haired people:
    Chamomile hair rinse. Purchase from a health food store or gather from your herb garden or nursery ¼ cup of chamomile flowers. Place them in a bowl. Pour 2 cups of boiling water over them. Allow to cool; strain and use.
    Rhubarb hair rinse. Purchase fresh (preferably organic) rhubarb from your local store. Chop into small pieces until you

have filled ¼ cup. Place it in a bowl. Pour 2 cups of boiling water over it. Allow to cool; strain and use.

- For women with naturally dark hair, these rinses have proven effective at adding highlights and color.

    Cinnamon hair rinse. Break three cinnamon sticks into small sections. Place them in a bowl. Pour 2 cups of boiling water over them. Allow to cool; strain and use.

    Lavender hair rinse. Use ¼ cup of lavender. Place it in a bowl. Pour 2 cups of boiling water over it. Allow to cool; strain and use.

    Sage hair rinse. Use ¼ cup of sage. Place it in a bowl. Pour 2 cups of boiling water over it. Allow to cool; strain and use.

- For red highlights:

    Hibiscus flowers. An especially excellent highlighting rinse for people desiring red highlights can be made from either a hibiscus flower–containing tea (purchased from a health food store) or dry hibiscus flowers. Bring 2 to 3 cups of water to a boil and pour it in a bowl; put in the flowers or tea. Allow the mixture to steep until the water reaches the desired shade. It is a good idea to use this rinse the first time in a lighter shade, which can be achieved by adding an extra cup or two of water; if desired, you can always make your hair darker with a second application.

RESOURCES

Mountain Light Henna Gray

Lotus Brands, Inc.
Box 325
Twin Lakes WI 53181
(414)889-8561

Schwarzkopf, Inc.

5701 Buckingham Parkway, Suite E
Culver City CA 90230
(800)234-4672

VitaWave

7131 Owensmouth Avenue, Suite 94D
Canoga Park CA 91303
(818)886-3808

Part VI

NINE TO FIVE

---

43. THE ALL-AMERICAN ROAD RACE . . . HOLD YOUR BREATH!

The concentration of hazardous chemicals from car exhaust is two to four times higher *inside* your car than outside.[1]

You somehow survive bumper-to-bumper traffic, talk-show zealots, tickets, drunk drivers, insurance premiums, and the noxious haze one hundred eighty million cars in this country spew out. But you're still not home free. The chemicals you breathe while driving in your car are hazardous to your health.

DID YOU KNOW:

- Vehicles in slow traffic (rush hour) have high concentrations of pollutants inside.[2]
- Vehicles in winter, with the windows up, have higher toxic concentrations than in summer.[3]

- A tuned car emits forty percent less hydrocarbons and fifty percent less carbon monoxide while providing you forty percent better gas mileage.[4]

Don't Get Stuck in Back of the Bus!

Exposure to diesel exhaust increases lung tumors and decreases learning ability and resistance to infections in experimental animals.[5]

Watch Your MPH—Most Potent Hazards

An EPA study found toluene, ethylene dibromide, xylene, ethylene dichloride, and benzene inside cars at levels two to four times higher than outdoors.[6] These chemicals are skin, lung, and eye irritants. Some cause headaches, fatigue, and cancer.[7] Did you say, "Fill'er up?"

SIMPLE THINGS TO DO

- Roll down your windows.
- Buy a car air filter. It plugs into your cigarette lighter. Finally, a use for that thing!
- Don't use products containing toxic chemicals to clean your car.
- Use gas pumps with vapor capture devices. Ask your local service station to install them if yours doesn't have them.
- Time your commutes for off-traffic hours. Many employers encourage this.
- Keep your car tuned.
- Some cars now provide built-in air filters. Ask your car dealer about these.
- Walk or ride a bike.
- If you're really serious, consider purchasing an alternative fuel vehicle.

RESOURCES

Air Filters

AllerMed

31 Steel Road
Wylie TX 75098
(214)442-4898

E.L. Foust Co. Inc.

P.O. Box 105
Elmhurst IL 60126
(800)225-9549

Alternative Fuel Vehicles

Electro-Automotive

P.O. Box 1113-GK
Fenton CA 95018
(408)429-1989

Green Motor Works

5228 Vineland Avenue
North Hollywood CA 91601
(818)766-3800

Gas Conversion Information

Western Propane Gas Association

7844 Madison Avenue
Fair Oaks CA 95628
(916)962-2280

44. YOU CAN'T GET THAT RAISE . . . IF YOU'RE NOT ALIVE

The chemical bonus you don't need . . .

OFFICE POLLUTION SOURCES

Source	Pollutant	Health Hazard
Particleboard shelving and furniture, plywood	Formaldehyde	Eye and skin irritation. Cancer.[1,2,3]
Glues	Toluene	Nerve damage. Birth defects. Headaches. Fatigue.[4]
Carpet backing	4-PC	Decreased immunity. Headaches. Fatigue. Chemical sensitivity.[5]
Dry copiers	Ozone	Lung irritation. Allergies.
Electrical devices, power junction boxes, computer terminals, microwave ovens, radiant heating, high tension wires and power substations	EMFs	Eye irritation. Cancer. Possibly birth defects.[6,7]
Permanent ink markers and pens	Xylene	Irritation. Nerve damage. Headaches.[8]
Insulation, ceiling and floor tiles	Asbestos	Cancer.
Pipes, lighting fixtures, upholstery, wall covering	Vinyl chloride	Irritation. Cancer.

Gimme a "Coffee" Break

The next time you grab that cup of java, you might want to know:

- Pesticides are sprayed on coffee crops.
- Hexane, which causes nerve damage, and methylene chloride, which causes cancer, are used to decaffeinate coffee.
- Dioxin, which causes cancer, leaches from bleached white coffee.
- Styrene leaches into coffee from polystyrene cups.

How about a mug of herbal tea?

SIMPLE THINGS TO DO

- Make sure the vents for your office air circulation system are open.
- Make sure the air circulation system is on during work hours.
- Talk to your boss or the building manager and find out when the building's system and ducts were last cleaned.
- Raise a ruckus if your boss puts you next to a copy machine or near a lab. If not properly vented, both can expose you to off-gassing chemicals.
- Use nontoxic glues, typewriter correction fluids, adhesives, and other office supplies.
- You might have to become a diplomat overnight, but ask your boss or building manager to use safer alternatives for pest control and cleaning. Most should be only too happy to help. It's their health too!
- While you have your boss's ear, why not recommend hardwood furniture and shelving over particleboard products?
- While hardwood or natural linoleum floors would be best, most offices are carpeted. Make sure if new carpeting is installed that it is done over the weekend, it is steam cleaned without detergents and solvents to pick up chemical residues, and a sealant is applied (see Chapter 5).

- Bring your own coffee mug—you'll save waste and not be drinking plastic.
- Use unbleached coffee filters or buy a coffeemaker that uses none.
- Ask the office manager to buy organic coffee.
- Buy a portable air filter for your car. Plug it in at your desk with the converter unit (see Chapter 43).
- Install a tinted radiation screen on your computer terminal. Tell your boss it eases eye strain and increases productivity (see Chapter 8).

RESOURCES

Least Toxic Paper Products

Conservatree Paper Company

10 Lombard St., Suite 250
San Francisco CA 94111
(415)433-1000

Earth Care Paper Co.

100 S. Baldwin
Madison WI 53703
(608)256-5522

Nontoxic Office Supplies

CHIP Distribution

P.O. Box 704
Manhattan Beach CA 90266
(310)545-5928

Seventh Generation

10 Farrell St.
South Burlington VT 05403
(800)456-1177

Worker Safety

National Institute for Occupational Safety and Health, Hazard Section

4676 Columbia Parkway
Cincinnati OH 45226
(513)684-2707

Environmental Protection Agency

401 M Street S.W.
Washington DC 20460

Right-to-know hotline: (800)535-0202

Part VII

BIG BROTHER'S WATCHING OVER YOU—WHO'S WATCHING OVER BIG BROTHER?

45. SAFE? WHO'S KIDDING WHO?

"As taxpayers we spend at least $828 million a year on government agencies employing over 20,000 people who are supposed to protect us from chemical hazards. Yet experts tell us much of our water isn't fit to drink, chemical dumps threaten our towns and rivers, our workplaces are filled with hazardous substances, and even our food contains untested, possibly unsafe, chemicals."

—EDWARD BERGIN AND RONALD
GRANDON[1]

You walk into the cocktail party a little apprehensive. It's in the Watergate, after all. The party invitation caught your curiosity: "G. Gordon Liddy and Colonel Oliver North invite you to a reception in honor of the public health contributions made by the tobacco and chemical industries," with "*not* printed on recycled paper" at the bottom.

Immediately to your right stand three goons who look like escaped mutants from *American Gladiators*. You're hungry. Nervously, you make your way to the hors d'oeuvres. Diet sodas featuring aspartame, Twinkies loaded with hydrogenated oil, a large crystal bowl filled with generic brand cigarettes, and a casserole dish of Prozac. You're not hungry. Three women sit against the far wall, advertisements for silicon breast implants, but they're gray, silent, and don't look well. You feel a shiver down your back. "Where am I?" Suddenly, someone taps you on the shoulder. "Can I get you a drink?" You jump but somehow manage to warily turn around—could this be Rush Limbaugh in drag?! Instinctively you look at your shaking hand, still clutching the crumpled invitation. You frantically flip it over, and look at the front—a picture of Laurence Olivier maniacally drilling Dustin Hoffman's teeth with a dentist bit; the caption reads, "Is It Safe?" You scream! You wake up. It is only a bad dream . . . or is it?

They Said It Was Safe

- DDT, PCBs, chlordane, kepone, asbestos, silicone breast implants, and leaded gasoline were all once proclaimed safe by government and industry, but later banned due to adverse health effects including cancer, nerve damage, and birth defects.
- Eighty percent of the industrial chemicals used today have had no toxicity testing.[2]
- While meat is one of the greatest sources of pesticide exposure in your diet,[3] the United States Department of Agriculture, responsible for food safety, tests only one out of every two hundred and fifty thousand slaughtered animals for toxic residues.[4]
- Even after being shown to cause cancer, diethylstilbestrol (DES), which causes rare vaginal cancers in women, was used for some forty years to hasten the weight gain of cattle. It was found at levels in the food supply known to cause cancer in rodents. Today, DES has been replaced by other cancer-causing growth stimulants which, for all practical purposes, are impossible to monitor in the meat supply.
- Chlordane was used for years in our homes to kill termites.

Velsicol Chemical, which makes it, withheld reports showing it caused cancer in animals.[5,6,7,8]

- Ignoring reports that the weed-killing chemical molinate causes harm to men's reproductive systems, California approved the continued use of the herbicide in rice fields.[9]

- Two scientists responsible for establishing "safe limits" for fifty-two chemicals in the workplace worked for Dow and DuPont. Many of the chemicals were also manufactured by Dow and DuPont.[10]

- Monsanto's medical director, while being cross-examined in a toxic chemical-related lawsuit, conceded under oath that researchers who conducted an important Monsanto cancer death study in 1983 knowingly fudged the data to equalize the death rates in "exposed" and "unexposed" workers. This suspect study was used by industry for years to trivialize risks associated with dioxins.[11]

- Millions of American children wore nightclothes treated with the fire retardant Tris, a powerful cancer-causing agent. It required some two years before the government acted to ban the chemical. Thousands of children are likely to contract cancer as a result.[12] U.S. manufacturers were allowed to dump Tris-treated sleepwear on the international market.

The Fox Watching the Hen House—and Getting Paid *for It!!*

Industrial Bio-Test Laboratories (IBT) safety-tested food additives, pesticides, and drugs for companies seeking government approvals. Hundreds of government approvals were given for pesticides, drugs, and food additives based on IBT information.[13] Then . . .

"IBT . . . faced with a federal investigation . . . for fraud and submission of questionable test data, destroyed files dealing with toxicological and carcinogenicity testing of thousands of federally approved products, including drugs, pesticides, food additives and industrial chemicals. The president of the company . . . admitted . . . at least four unidentified major pesticide manufacturers were aware of this fraud when they submitted the test data in product applications. In spite of the questionable validity of tests documenting their safety, the government refused to take these chemicals off the market."

—SAMUEL EPSTEIN, M.D,
The Politics of Cancer

We Can't Always Wait for Uncle Sam

- Courageous efforts, like that of Love Canal resident Lois Gibbs, finally moved Congress to pass a law to clean up hazardous waste dumps.[14]
- The Natural Resources Defense Council has fought and won legal suits against our own government for safer air, water, and food.[15]
- We suffered one hundred thousand deaths a year from workplace injuries before Congress passed the Occupational Safety and Health Act.[16]
- Millions of birds had to die and Rachel Carson had to write *Silent Spring* before laws to control hazardous pesticides were enacted.
- Cesar Chavez endured covert investigations by the FBI while he used hunger strikes and boycotts to bring the plight of pesticide-exposed farm workers to public attention.

SIMPLE THINGS TO DO

- Buy least toxic alternatives.
- Educate yourself (see Chapter 50).
- Support legitimate boycotts of unsafe products.
- Whenever possible, avoid buying products made by known corporate polluters.
- Help the tireless, undermanned, underfinanced, often unthanked groups that constantly fight, unseen, for your and your family's environmental health.

RESOURCES

Cancer Prevention Coalition
520 North Michigan Avenue, Suite 410
Chicago IL 60611
(312)467-0600

Citizen Action
800 Custer Street, Suite 6
Evanston IL 60202
(847)332-1776

Citizen's Clearinghouse for Hazardous Wastes
P.O. Box 6806
Falls Church VA 22040
(703)237-CCHW

Common Cause
2030 M St. N.W.
Washington DC 20036
(202)833-1200

Environmental Defense Fund
257 Park Avenue South
New York NY 10010
(212)505-2100

Greenpeace
1436 U St. N.W.
Washington DC 20009
(202)462-1177
Internet address: http://www.greenpeace.org/

National Coalition Against Misuse of Pesticides
701 E Street S.E.
Washington DC 20003
(202)543-5450
(202)543-4791 (Fax)
e-mail: NCAMP@igc.apc.org

Natural Resources Defense Council

40 West 20th St.
New York NY 10011
(212)727-2700

The Rachel Carson Council

8940 Jones Mill Road
Chevy Chase MD 20815
(301)652-1877

United Farm Workers

P.O. Box 62
Keene CA 93531
(805)822-5571

46. YOU CAN HAVE IT, I DON'T WANT IT

"Pesticides banned in the United States because they can cause cancer, birth defects and brain damage are exported to foreign countries that have less stringent environmental laws. One study found in just a three-month period nearly sixteen million pounds of these poisons were shipped—that's more than three tons per hour."

—FOUNDATION FOR ADVANCEMENTS
IN SCIENCE AND EDUCATION[1]

The Golden Rule, Redefined

Everyone has a pesky neighbor who makes us shake our head and chuckle under our breath. Joe's one. Maybe it's his morning jaunts to fetch the paper, sporting a three-day stubble, in pajamas six inches above his ankles. Or the mushy apples he pawns off to the kids on Halloween. Anyway, the only thing you say to him all year is "thanks" for a Christmas fruitcake you use for rat bait. But Joe has a problem. Cockroaches and ants are overrunning his house, and his wife has him sleeping on the porch until they're gone. He grudgingly wanders in the basement and digs out an old bug spray. He sprays it everywhere. His grass, trees, and rosebushes are all shriveled, and the critters that got away are in your house now, but he's sleeping in his bed again. Joe needs some money for the local nursery, so he cons you into buying the bug spray for half price. It's a deal, he tells you. But he conveniently forgets to tell you it's been banned for the last ten years. You spray your home. Your whole family gets sick. How do you feel about Joe now? Well, don't look too far, because some United States chemical companies are playing the role of your quirky neighbor Joe.[2]

American chemical manufacturers routinely export to foreign countries pesticides that have been banned in the United States. The EPA has no authority to stop them.[3] In other words, the golden rule, as redefined by exporters of United States–banned pesticides, is that those who have the gold rule. And we wonder what's gone wrong with American foreign policy?

Did You Know:

- Approximately three million cases of pesticide poisoning occur annually with over two hundred thousand deaths.[4]
- While eighty percent of pesticides and other agricultural chemicals are used in developed countries, more than ninety-nine percent of all deaths from pesticide poisoning occur in developing nations.[5]
- Indonesia banned fifty-seven pesticides, many imported from the United States, because they provided no increased crop yields, but did increase environmental problems.[6]
- From March through May in 1990, over one hundred twenty million pounds of pesticides were exported from the United States. Over twelve million pounds classified as extremely toxic, including banned cancer-causing chemicals such as chlordane, mirex, and heptachlor, were sent overseas. Some six million pounds, in total, either cause cancer or birth defects.[7,8]
- Much of the food imported into the United States is contami-

nated with pesticides banned in the United States because they cause cancer, nerve damage, and birth defects.[9] When contaminated foods return to American consumers, this is called the "circle of poison."

Code Name . . . Deceit

Under the guise of "trade secrets," pesticide manufacturers may delete their names from export documents and use instead the generic term "order." In a study of a three-month period of United States Custom records a company using the generic term "Order, St. Louis, MO" exported over twenty million pounds of pesticides. The only exporter listed in custom records as being from St. Louis during that period was Monsanto. Disclosure loopholes make it possible to export virtually any pesticide, regardless of hazard—covertly and anonymously.[10]

SIMPLE THINGS TO DO

- Buy organic fruits and vegetables (see Chapter 24).
- Avoid nonorganic imported fruits, vegetables, or meats.
- Choose in-season produce to avoid imported foods.
- Write your elected representatives insisting they support legislation outlawing the exporting of unsafe pesticides.
- Boycott companies and products that profit from exporting dangerous pesticides.

RESOURCES

Foundation for Advancements in Science and Education

4801 Wilshire Blvd., Suite 215
Los Angeles CA 90010
(213)937-9911

A clearinghouse for reports on pesticide exports.

47. A MAN NAMED DELANEY

You probably never met him, shook his hand, shared a joke, or for that matter had his mobile phone number. But a man named James Delaney probably has done more for your family's health than anyone since an Englishman invented the modern toilet.

The 1958 federal Food, Drug, and Cosmetic Act contains a simple clause written by Congressman Delaney (D-NY) stating that pesticides "found to induce cancer when ingested by man or animal" are not safe and cannot be allowed in processed food at *any* level. While the law permits the EPA to allow cancer-causing pesticides to be sprayed on crops (raw oranges, potatoes, apples, and grapes), residues of cancer-causing pesticides are strictly prohibited by the Delaney Clause in *any* processed foods at any level. This means apple sauce, juices, cereals, and frozen foods.

We are bombarded with low levels of toxic chemicals every day. Industry proponents claim these levels are so low they can't hurt you.[1] Maybe no single, low-level exposure kills, but the sum total increases your toxic dose to a level never seen before in history. Has one of these industry proponents ever listed all the chemicals you are exposed to in a single day, then looked you in the eye and told you the combined impact on your health is zilch? Don't think so. If he did, he'd probably start stuffing letters for Greenpeace. The Delaney Clause eliminates a major source of cancer-causing chemicals. It reduces our dose. It reduces our risk.

DID YOU KNOW:

- Animal studies used to determine cancer look only at a single chemical at a time. In the real world, people are exposed to many chemicals at once. Current tests may not be tough enough— cancer is on the rise.[2]
- The Delaney Clause is scientifically sound—how do you figure

a "safe" level for a chemical that causes cancer at every dose tested? Who wants to guess?

- If pesticide use was cut in half, food cost would rise less than one percent, while the nation would save as much as ten billion dollars a year in decreased environmental damage and regulatory and medical costs.[3]
- The biggest lie: pesticides are necessary to grow our food. They might be necessary to company profits, but there has never been an adequate industry investigation of successful farming techniques that eliminate toxic chemicals while improving crop yields and soil quality.[4]

Your Friend the Delaney Clause Is Being Sliced and Diced

Since 1958, laboratories have learned how to measure smaller amounts of chemicals in food. They now regularly find toxic pesticides in processed foods in clear violation of the Delaney Clause. What's industry's answer? You got it. *Kill Delaney!*

An army of well-funded industry "experts," lawyers, and lobbyists, touting the benefits of small amounts of cancer-causing chemicals in your food, finally persuaded the Bush Administration and the EPA in 1988 to adopt the "negligible risk" policy—small amounts of cancer-causing pesticides in processed food were acceptable.

Score One for the Good Guys . . .

The Natural Resources Defense Council, Public Citizen, and other groups challenged EPA's new "negligible risk" policy. The United States Court of Appeals ruled that "if pesticides which concentrate in processed foods induce cancer in humans or animals, they render the food adulterated and must be prohibited."[5,6]

It's Not Over Till It's Over . . .

Industry is still trying to eliminate Delaney. They must be using that guy who told Congress nicotine wasn't addictive.

SIMPLE THINGS TO DO

Demand that your elected officials:
- Pass legislation to phase out all cancer-causing pesticides from processed and raw foods.
- Protect the Delaney Clause and strengthen it.
- Require new chemicals to be fully tested for all health effects.
- Encourage the use of proven nontoxic alternative methods for growing food.
- Join groups fighting to protect Delaney, clean up the food supply, and protect your health.

RESOURCES

National Coalition Against the Misuse of Pesticides
530 701 E Street S.E.
Washington DC 20003
(202)543-5450
(202)543-4791 (Fax)
e-mail:
NCAMP@ igc.apc.org

Natural Resources Defense Council
40 West 20th St.
New York NY 10011
(212)727-2700

48. FOLLOW THE MONEY

Not long ago I (David Steinman) received an anonymous letter from a former clerical employee of Ketchum Communications, a major public relations firm. At the firm, the writer said he or she participated in the compilation of promotional materials for the California Raisin Advisory Board (CALRAB). The writer reported that CALRAB was uneasy when I revealed in my book *Diet for a Poisoned Planet* that raisins are sprayed with a pesticide containing DDT—this, even in the nineties, some twenty years after most Americans thought that DDT was banned by the government and had disappeared from the food supply. The writer said he or she decided to write me because he or she was angry with what he or she felt was Ketchum's effort to promote its client's interests by mounting a campaign to discredit my writings on toxins in food and household products without ever considering the merits of my position.

In the letter the writer reports that the firm tracked down all my scheduled television talk show appearances during a certain period of time and called up the producer of each show to raise doubts about my credibility or demand equal time for the food growers. It was their plan, he or she believed, to paint me as an extreme radical.

"Because the data you used was largely government data, Ketchum was in a quandary about how to rebut the toxicity of the raisin," he or she wrote. "They hired between three and five independent laboratory services to discredit your reporting techniques, the way you came to your conclusions, and whatever else they could attack. . . . The only concern was that your book not do financial damage to CALRAB, as the alar scare damaged apple growers. . . ."   —Ex-Ketchum Communications Staffer, 1992

Although I was unable to contact the writer to question him or her directly, he or she provided documentation of these charges that appeared to be genuine.

ABC Chemical Company is interviewing for a senior research chemist. Bill sits nervously in a row of chairs with other hopeful applicants. When it is his turn, he discusses his Ph.D., work at MIT, and nomination for a Nobel prize in chemistry. He does a good job. He answers questions honestly. The last applicant enters the waiting area as Bill returns. They are old college friends. Bill decides to wait to chat with his old friend. A few minutes later, the last applicant emerges from his interview. Bill anxiously asks, "How did it go?"

"OK," he says. "They asked me, if I had to test the effects of chemical X on population Y, how would I design a study?"

"Me too," Bill says. "What did you say?"

" 'What results do you want?' " he says.

"You said that?" Bill says. "That isn't science. It isn't even ethical."

"I got the job."

This is no joke. While there are many conscientious people in government and private industry, a few scientists, business managers, advertising executives, and public officials, under financial pressure or out of political and scientific prejudice, forget their public trust and foist upon us chemicals and drugs that threaten our health both now and forty years from now.

DID YOU KNOW:

- Public relations firms, such as Ketchum Communications and Hill and Knowlton, are paid more than $75 million annually to promote "greenwashing," the concept that there are only "trivial" health effects for a wide range of chemical pollutants.[1] It all comes out "green" in the wash.

- Usually, these so-called "objective" and "impartial" sources sport names like the Information Council for National Safety, Motherhood, and Apple Pie,[2] according to environmental columnist Donella Meadows.

- In a television ad, a meadow filled with wildflowers and litter is being cleaned up by children who are using plastic bags that are advertised as biodegradable, notes businessman and ecologist Paul Hawken. Native Americans look on approvingly. In fact, these bags were shown to be *not* biodegradable. The advertisement's sponsor, Mobil Oil, was sued in several states for this ad.[3]

- Donella Meadows, environmental columnist, reports that when the EPA published a small book providing information on how to be environmentally responsible, it was quickly canceled. "Why? Because it suggested that you can reduce hazardous chemicals in your house by using soap flakes instead of laundry detergent, vinegar to clean glass, cedar chips for mothballs, boric acid to repel ants, and boiling water instead of commercial drain cleaner."[4] The publication was labeled as irresponsible by Procter & Gamble, manufacturer of many cleaning products, claiming that consumers who followed the EPA's make-your-own advice could be injured. Is P&G trying to clean up your home *and your mind?*

- "When Chairman Rawl of Exxon warns us that if we don't open up the last and largest wildlife refuge in the United States to oil drilling and exploration, 'the entire nation will forfeit . . . substantial economic benefits,' we are not being schooled in classical economics, but in Exxonian economics," notes Hawken. He goes on to add that ceiling insulation and double-glazed windows will produce far more oil than the Arctic National Wildlife Refuge at its most optimistic projections, "at about one-twentieth the cost."[5]

- One of the widely cited "experts" in the media on health and the environment is Elizabeth Whelan, of the American Council on Science and Health (ACSH). Whelan often relies on the false-dilemma theory of persuasion. Yes, water chlorination causes cancer, she says in one of her books, but without it, many more people would die of infectious disease. This is all true. Her conclusion: drink chlorinated water and stop complaining! She does not mention using a water filter. According to Whelan, pesticides and industrial pollutants are trivial risks. But what is not revealed is that ACSH receives large sums of money from a list of companies that reads like a who's who of corporate polluters, including Dow Chemical Canada, Exxon Corporation, Monsanto,

and Union Carbide—according to the group's own documents.
- Bovine growth hormone (BGH), used to increase cows' milk production, poses a potential risk for colon cancer.[6] It was banned in the European community. But here in the United States, BGH has become something of its own "sacred cow." FDA officials have gone so far as to prohibit independent dairy producers and distributors from using "hormone-free" labels on milk from cows raised without BGH, stating labeling would be false and illegal under federal law, as milk from treated cows, they say, is "virtually the same" as that from untreated animals. However, some states have passed their own legislation permitting such labeling. So how did BGH get into American dairy products, without any labeling, when its use internationally has been prohibited? Congressmen David R. Obey, D-Wisconsin, and George E. Brown, Jr., D-California, as well as independent representative Bernie Sanders of Vermont, think they have the answer. They note that several key administrative employees at the FDA who were responsible for that agency's formal position on the use of BGH were formerly closely associated with Monsanto. Although FDA spokesman Jim O'Hara contends that allegations of conflict of interest are "without any basis," the Government Accounting Office was asked by the congressmen to launch an investigation.[7]
- Samuel S. Epstein, M.D., a leading cancer expert, tells how a chemical is given a "clean bill of health": In 1971, Dow published information, based on its own tests of 2,4-D, a widely used lawn weed killer, that claimed testing in rats demonstrated it was not a cause of birth defects. However, Dow redefined birth defects to include only those that were fatal, Epstein notes. Thus, under this criteria, deformities, including missing limbs, were not considered to be birth defects. Data from the study, when carefully reviewed, indicated the occurrence of extensive birth defects.[8]

SIMPLE THINGS TO DO

- Understand that science and public policy it engenders is, at its best, a democratic process. Anybody can participate if they have something worthwhile to say. Science is a violent public argument. It is what people believe. It does not matter if they have a Ph.D. or M.D. or any other alphabet after their name. Such degrees do not automatically confer competent judgment, wisdom, public policy sense, or fairness. These qualities are earned. When someone has to assert their degree as proof of their superior wisdom, all they are really saying is they have run out of steam and must now resort to attacks no matter which side of the argument they are on.
- Never accept a scientific study or public statement at face value.
- Never leap to conclusions based on a single study or statement.
- Always find out who funded the study or is paying the salary of the spokesperson. This cuts both ways. Environmentalists and polluters deserve equal scrutiny.
- Develop a healthy skepticism. Be wary of greenwashing.
- Learn how so-called objective experimental studies can be flawed.[9]

RESOURCES

PR Watch

3318 Gregory St.
Madison WI 53711
(608)233-3346
Fax: (608)238-2236

Subscribe to PR Watch *to get the inside story on "greenwashing." Also write for information on media training for activists and other related issues.*

United States General Accounting Office (GAO)

P.O. Box 6015

Gaithersburg MD 20884-6015

(202)512-6000

Fax: (301)258-4066

The GAO produces a wide range of documents on public and private areas of interest, including health and the environment, that attempt to expose conflicts of interest and coverups. Get on their document mailing list. Their publications are free.

49. ROCK THE VOTE

"When these PACs give money, they expect something in return rather than good government."

—SENATOR ROBERT DOLE, KANSAS

"You can't buy a congressman for $5,000. But you can buy his vote. It's done on a regular basis."

—REPRESENTATIVE THOMAS DOWNEY, NEW YORK

To industry spokespersons and their paid scientists who say that the doses of toxins to which all of us are being exposed are so low as to be meaningless, we simply say that the nation is in the midst of a cancer epidemic. More than one in three will be stricken. More than one in four men, women, and children will die from cancer.

Your vote counts. Elections matter. Were you one of the millions who voted in a Republican congress—only to discover that rather than conservatives, they are simply all too often fronts for corporate greed? They often operate as if what's good for corporate America is good for you. If they actually had integrity and were not just marching in lockstep, they'd fight for what the people who elected them want: reduced government waste, reduced deficit, reduced government, and increased protection of public health and the environment. If they were true conservatives, they'd do their accounting and find out, while it might cost a few corporate contributors some short-term profits, that billions and billions of dollars more could be saved in natural resources, energy, and health care costs if we stopped poisoning ourselves and our planet with toxic chemicals while we mortgage our country's soul to some guy in the Middle East. The fact that so few have broken ranks to think for themselves tells us they are marching to the same old Pied Piper.

In the first one hundred days of the Contract on America, coal company lawyers rewrote the clean air laws, and toxic chemical manufacturers rewrote the Clean Water Act.[1] If they'd had a few more days, one suspects the Mafia would have rewritten the crime bill.

Are you tired of being the last person to know that you have been transformed into an environmental guinea pig?

It is time to rock the vote.

DID YOU KNOW:

- The most antienvironmental and antipublic health voting bloc in Congress is the seventy-three new Republicans elected in November 1994. Their average League of Conservation Voters (LCV) score is three percent (with one hundred percent being perfect). Sixty-one of the seventy-three scored an absolute zero.[2]
- Democrats are not always proenvironment and propublic health, either. A new caucus of twenty-three Democratic members has made dismantling environmental protection a priority.[3]
- If our representatives had been working to make our economy as energy-efficient as that of Sweden or Japan, "we would have been spending two hundred billion dollars a year *less* in energy costs during the past decade, an amount equal to the average annual budget deficit incurred by the federal government."[4]
- If pollution laws were put into effect, manufacturers would have the incentive to market cars which already exist and get nearly

ninety-eight miles per gallon, notes Paul Hawken. Cars on the drawing board that can get as high as two hundred miles per gallon could become reality tomorrow.[5]

SIMPLE THINGS TO DO

- Be informed about the voting records of your representatives. Join the League of Conservation Voters and get that organization's Congressional National Environmental Scorecard. State by state, it's easy to find out how your representatives have voted on key health and environmental legislative bills.
- Call the President at (202)456-1111 or write to 1600 Pennsylvania Avenue, Washington DC 20500.
- Obtain a copy of the telephone directories for the Senate and House of Representatives from the Government Printing Office. Become familiar with their staff members and district representatives.
- Call your senator or congressional representative at (202)224-3121. Write your senator at the United States Senate, Washington DC 20510. Write your congressional representative at the United States House of Representatives, Washington DC 20515.
- Contact environmental legislative hotlines to keep regularly updated.

RESOURCES

Congressional Telephone Directories

Government Printing Office
P.O. Box 37000
Washington DC 20013-7000
(202)789-0420

Environmental Legislative Scorecard

League of Conservation Voters (LCV)
1707 L St. N.W., Suite 750
Washington DC 20036
(202)785-8638
Fax: (202)835-0491

Join the LCV and receive its annual Congressional National Environmental Scorecard. Receive much more frequent updates through the Internet at http://www.econet.apc.org/lcv/scorecard.html.

Environmental Hot Lines

Clean Water Network

1350 New York Avenue N.W., Suite 300
Washington DC 20005
(202)624-9357

Use the network's action hotline. Call (202) 624-9339.

National Audubon Society

700 Broadway
New York NY 10003
(800)274-4201
(212)979-3000

Use the action hotline. Call (800) 659-2622.

National Wildlife Federation

1400 16th Street N.W.
Washington DC 20036
(202)797-6800

Use the action hotline. Call (202) 797-6655.

Sierra Club

730 Polk St.
San Francisco CA 94109
(415)776-2211

Use the action hotline. Call (202) 675-2394.

Internet address: http://www.sierraclub.org

Part VIII

AND TO ADD TO ALL THAT

———————— ✎ ————————

50. THROW THE BOOK AT IT!

"First and foremost, we must protect the minds and bodies of children from the ravages of pollution. We must develop environmental youth education programs that teach the words, concepts, the fundamentals of ecology. We need to tell them the truth. This is our future, it's theirs."

—TOM CRUISE[1]

Following is suggested reading for the many topics covered in this book. Other books of possible interest are mentioned in the reference notes.

2. If You Don't Know the Words, You Can't Sing the Tune

Cry Out: An Illustrated Guide to What You Can Do to Save the Earth

The Alley Foundation, 1990, Beverly Hills, Cal.

A color booklet for children featuring environmental and health problems and solutions. Complete illustrated glossary. Free: (213)932-7968.

The New American Medical Dictionary

edited by Robert Rothenberg, M.D.
Signet Books, 1990, New York.

A pocket guide for defining medical terms.

3. Everybody's Talkin'

The Amazing Environmental Organization Web Directory

Internet address: http://www.web directory.com/

A good place to begin. This resource serves as a yellow pages of green Web sites.

Enviro Web

Internet address: http://www.envirolink.org/

A comprehensive collection of environmental information. Is the mother of environmental Internet sites. Links to hundreds of environmental alerts, groups, businesses, and educational resources.

Eco Net

Internet address: http://econet.apc.org/econet/

Maintained by San Francisco's Institute for Global Communications. Is the world's first major environmental computer network. Carries local, national, and international environmental campaigns. E-Mail: econet-info@econet.apc.org.

Public Interest Research Groups

Internet address: http://www.igc.apc.org/pirg/

Inspired by Ralph Nader, founded by students, is the largest network of grass-roots environmental and consumer groups containing information on toxins, pesticides, recycling, clean air and water.

Fifty Simple Things You Can Do to Save the Earth

by The EarthWorks Group
Earthworks Press, 1989, Berkeley, Cal.

Read it, use it. It's fun and important.

Heaven Is Under Our Feet

by Don Henley and David Marsh
Longmeadow Press, 1991, Stamford, Conn.

A wonderful anthology of environmental essays from leading thinkers of our time, from past Presidents, environmentalists, artists, authors, and others.

4. Clean House

The Non-Toxic Home

by Debra Lynn Dadd
Jeremy Tarcher, Inc., 1986, Los Angeles.

A classic book on home toxic hazards and simple, earthy solutions.

5. Pull the Rug Out

Toxic Carpet III

by Glenn Beebe
Beebe, 1991, Cincinnati.

A moving and informative narrative of a family decimated by toxins from carpet and their fight to overcome. Has detailed information on carpet hazards and chemistry.

7. Paint Your Wagon

Artists Beware!

by Dr. Michael McCann
Lyons on Burford, 1992, New York.

Household Solvent Products: A Shelf Survey with Laboratory Analysis

by Westat Inc. and Midwest Research Institute
Office of Toxic Substances, US EPA, 1987, Washington, D.C.

A survey of some of the most common solvents in the home and office.

8. Wired!

Biological Effects of Power Frequency Electric and Magnetic Fields

Government Printing Office, #052-003-01152-2, Washington, D.C.

An informative review of some of the health hazards and sources of EMFs.

Currents of Death: Power Lines, Computer Terminals and the Attempt to Cover Up Their Threat to Your Health

by Paul Brodeur
Little, Brown and Company, 1995, Boston.

A controversial and ground-breaking book on the health effects of electromagnetic fields and industry/governments efforts to hide these.

9. Are You Glowing in the Dark?

United States Map of Geographical Areas with Potentially High Radon Levels

U.S. Environmental Protection Agency
401 M Street S.W.
Washington, D.C. 20460

All About Radiation

by L. Ron Hubbard
Bridge Publications, 1979, Los Angeles.

A unique and forward-looking book on the effects of radiation. First published in 1957, it is hauntingly accurate in its predictions, and uplifting in its solutions.

Radon: A Homeowner's Guide to Detection and Control

by Bernard Cohen and the editors of *Consumer Reports*.

A homeowner's user's manual for detection and control of Radon.

10. Freeze 'Em, Zap 'Em

Basic Guide to Pesticides

by Shirley A. Briggs and Rachel Carson Council
Hemisphere Publishing, 1992, Washington, D.C.

13. Attack of the Killer House . . . Building It Better

Healthful Houses: How to Design and Build Your Own

by Clint Goode
Guaranty Press, 1988, Lincoln, Va.

A classic book that gives architectural and construction details for building a healthy house.

The Healthy House

by John Brower
Carol Publishing, 1993, Secaucus, N.J.

A comprehensive, easy-to-read, thoroughly documented book on toxic home hazards and solutions with an extensive resource section.

16. Just Say No!

Physicians' Desk Reference (PDR)

Edward Barnhart, Publisher
Medical Economics Company, 1995, Oradell, N.J.

If you ever take a drug, you want this comprehensive review of all side effects in your home. Most doctors have one; you'll probably end up reading it more often.

Prescription Drugs and Their Side Effects

by Edward Stern
Grosset & Dunlap, 1978, New York.

A simple guide to help you know the side effects of the most common drugs.

The Truth About Drugs

by John Duff and Gene Chill
Bridge Publications, 1981, Los Angeles.

A unique description of drugs and the problems they create. Lists innovative alternatives.

17. What's Up, Doc?

Methods for Biological Monitoring: A Manual for Assessing Human Exposure to Hazardous Substances

by Theodore Kneip and John Crable
American Public Health Association, 1988, Washington, D.C.

A health professional's guide for tests to determine the harmful effects of chemicals.

Complete Home Medical Guide: Columbia College of Physicians

edited by Donald Tapley, M.D.
Crown Publishers, 1985, New York.

A comprehensive yet understandable layperson's guide to just about every major medical question from fevers to home poisonings.

The Role of the Primary Care Physician in Occupational and Environmental Medicine

by the National Research Council Institute of Medicine
National Academy Press, 1988, Washington, D.C.

A startling and eye-opening review of American physicians and their lack of training for diagnosing and treating chemically induced health problems.

19. Get Smart!

Is This Your Child?

by Doris Rapp, M.D.
William Morrow and Company, 1991, New York.

A best-selling answer to saving a hyperactive, problematic child without harmful drugs or therapies.

Pesticides in the Diets of Infants and Children

by the Committee on Pesticides in the Diets of Infants and Children
National Academy Press, 1993, Washington, D.C.

A milestone scientific review of the health effects of pesticides in the diet of children and infants.

Raising Toxic Free Kids

by Phillip Landrigan, M.D.

Why Your Child Is Hyperactive

by Benjamin Feingold
Random House, 1974, New York.

The ground-breaking book that started an entire new look at the chemicals and additives in food and their effect on children. Must reading for a historical perspective.

20. Don't Sweat It . . . Yes, Do!

Clear Body, Clear Mind

by L. Ron Hubbard
Bridge Publications, 1990, Los Angeles.

Details in simple, understandable terms a comprehensive detoxification program that has become the most scientifically proven and applauded means of ridding the body of toxic chemicals and drugs.

The Poisoned Womb

by John Elkington
Penguin Books, 1985, New York.

A startling account of the dangers of toxins to the new and unborn.

Silent Spring

by Rachel Carson
Houghton Mifflin Co., 1962, Boston.

The book that started an entire awareness of modern chemicals and their effect on the environment and Man.

22. You Are What You Eat—And Then Some

Diet for a New America

by John Robbins
Stillpoint Publishing, 1987, Walpole, N.H.

A compelling argument on health, environmental, and moral grounds for a diet rich in fruits, vegetables, and grains and void of fatty meats.

Monitoring Human Tissues for Toxic Substances

by Committee on National Monitoring of Human Tissues, Board on Environmental Studies and Toxicology, and Commission on Life Sciences
National Academy Press, 1991, Washington, D.C.

A scientific review of the toxic chemicals accumulating in humans today.

23. Save Your Waistline While Poisons Miss the Mark

Choose to Live

by Joseph Weissman, M.D.
Penguin Books, 1988, New York.

An original book covering the toxic hazards from a high-fat diet. Offers solutions.

The Safe Shopper's Bible

by David Steinman and Samuel S. Epstein, M.D.
Macmillan Press, 1995, New York.

If you want to shop for food or anything else while avoiding toxins and health hazards, add this to your grocery list, then take it shopping with you.

24. Eat It—Organic

Diet for a Poisoned Planet

by David Steinman
Ballantine Books, 1992, New York.

If you want to know what poisons are in your food and how to eat well and healthy while avoiding them, get this book.

Pesticide Alert

by Lawrie Mott and Karen Snyder
Sierra Books, 1987, San Francisco.

A comprehensive review of pesticides, their hazards, and where we are exposed to them.

The Way We Grow: Good Sense Solutions for Protecting Our Families From Pesticides in Food

by Anne Witte Garland
Berkley Publishing Group, 1994, New York.

Identifies pesticide and health hazards in diet and offers safe, simple solutions.

26. How Sweet It Isn't

Aspartame (Nutrasweet): Is It Safe??

by Harvey Roberts, M.D.
The Charles Press, 1990, Philadelphia.

An informative and revealing look into the dangers of this artificial sweetener.

The Bitter Truth About Artificial Sweeteners

by Dennis Remington, M.D., and Barbara Higa, R.D.
Vitality House, 1987, Provo, Utah.

One of the first books to disclose the hazards and shady approval process of artificial sweeteners. Cites numerous studies and scientific articles.

28. You Make Me So Excited . . .

Excitotoxins: The Taste That Kills

by Russell Blaylock, M.D.
Health Press, 1994, Santa Fe, N.M.

A startling, revealing book on the hazards of artificial sweeteners, MSG, and hydrolyzed vegetable protein. Buy this, read this, and you'll never buy them again.

In Bad Taste: The MSG Syndrome

by George Schwartz
Health Press, 1988, Santa Fe, N.M.

A revealing book on the hazards of MSG.

A Quick Guide to Food Safety

by Robert Goodman
Silvercat Publications, 1992, San Diego.

A simple, rudimentary guide to food safety.

33. I Have One Word for You—Plastic

The Green Consumer

by John Elkington, Julia Hailes, and Joel Makower
Penguin Books, 1990, New York.

Provides healthy, environmentally friendly solutions to modern consumer goods.

Wrapped in Plastics

by Jeanne Wirka
Environmental Action Foundation, 1988, Washington, D.C.

A keen look at the environmental and health costs of plastics.

34. Wax Your Car, Not Your Tummy

The Wax Coverup: What Consumers Aren't Told About Pesticides on Fresh Produce.

Americans for Safe Food: Center for Science and the Public Interest, Washington, D.C.

An expose on the waxing of foods, its hazards and regulatory disregard.

35. Snow White Has a Black Heart

Dying From Dioxin: A Citizen's Guide to Reclaiming Our Health and Rebuilding Democracy

by Lois Marie Gibbs
South End Press, 1995, Boston.

A comprehensive description of dioxin in the environment, its consequences on health, and the regulatory and industry coverups.

37. Voting at the Checkout Line

The Safe Shopper's Guide: A Consumer's Guide to Nontoxic Household Products, Cosmetics, and Food

by David Steinman and Samuel S. Epstein, M.D.
Macmillan, 1995, New York

The definitive safe-shopping guide. Rates thousands of major and alternative brand products.

38. Put a Pretty Face On

Natural Organic Hair and Skin Care

by Aubry Hampton
Organica Press, 1987, Tampa, Fla.

Hampton is a nationally known producer of fine cosmetics and body care products. He can afford to tell it like it is: After all, his products don't contain toxic chemicals.

Natural Beauty at Home

by Janice Cox
Henry Holt, 1994, New York.

This is one of the best books on making your own cosmetics and has more than two hundred recipes for your body, bath, and hair.

39. I Smell a Rat

Consumer's Dictionary of Cosmetic Ingredients

by Ruth Winter
Crown Publishers, 1989, New York.

A pocket guide to the chemicals you splash on yourself in the bathroom.

Health Hazard Information

by Julia Kendall
Environmental Protection Agency, 1991, Washington, D.C.

A regulatory review of scents and fragrances.

44. You Can't Get That Raise . . . If You're Not Alive

The Green Shalom Guide

edited by Naomi Friedman and Herman De Fischler
Greater Washington, D.C., Shomrei Adamah, Tacoma Park, MD.

A how-to manual for greening local Jewish synagogues, schools, offices.

EPA Journal: Indoor Air

United States Environmental Protection Agency
US EPA; 1993; 19(4): EPA 175-N-93-027, Washington, D.C.

A regulatory review of indoor air health hazards.

The Nontoxic Home and Office

by Debra Lynn Dadd
Jeremy Tarcher, Inc., 1992, Los Angeles.

Details toxic hazards in the home and office and offers simple solutions.

Workers With Multiple Chemical Sensitivity

by Mark Cullen, M.D.
Hanley and Belfus, 1987, Philadelphia.

A scientific review of an increasing modern illness from chemicals.

45. Safe? Who's Kidding Who?

How to Survive in Your Toxic Environment

by Edward Bergin and Ronald Grandon
Avon Books, 1984, New York.

An early, revealing look at the toxic hazards in modern life and industry and government coverups. Provides an action outline and resources.

Love Canal: My Story

by Lois Marie Gibbs
State University of New York Press, 1982, Albany, N.Y.

A story of a family's horror from toxic wastes and their courageous determination to survive.

Pesticides and Regulation: The Myth of Safety

by Bruce Jennings
California Senate Office of Research, 1991, Sacramento, Cal.

A positively revealing report on the hazards of pesticides and the lack of testing, education, and prevention of these by government.

Rating Corporate America

by Steven D. Lydenberg, Alice Tepper Marlin, Sean O'Brien Strub and the Council of Economic Priorities.
Addison-Wesley Publishing, 1986, Reading, Mass.

A guide for rating the social and environmental conscience of major corporations and their products. A must for an environmentally conscious investor.

Shopping for a Better World

The Council on Economic Opportunities, 1994, New York.

A comprehensive guide and rating system for environmentally friendly and unfriendly corporations and products. A shopper's guide to environmental responsibility.

46. You Can Have It, I Don't Want It

Exporting Banned and Hazardous Pesticides: A Preliminary Report

The Foundation for Advancements in Science and Education, 1991, Los Angeles.

A chilling and painstakingly factual documentation of American exports of toxic, hazardous pesticides. This report revealed for the first time its actual scope and pervasiveness.

Exporting Banned Pesticides: Fueling the Circle of Poison

by Sue Marquardt
Greenpeace, 1989, Washington, D.C.

Details the horrific practice of exporting toxins abroad that come back to us in imported foods.

47. A Man Named Delaney

EPA Journal: *The Delaney Clause Dilemma*

by Victor J. Kimm
United States Environmental Protection Agency, 1993, Washington,
D.C.

A regulatory view on the Delaney clause debate.

**Escape From the Pesticide Treadmill: Alternatives to Pesticides in
Developing Countries**

by Michael Hansen, Ph.D.
Institute for Consumer Policy Research: Consumers Union, 1987,
Mount Vernon, N.Y.

*Brilliant, innovative case studies on nonpesticide farming techniques that in-
crease crop yields and enhance soil conditions without the expense and hazards
of chemicals.*

NCAMP's Technical Report

National Coalition Against the Misuse of Pesticides, 1992, Washington,
D.C.

*A hard-line, no-nonsense report on the hazards of pesticides and current reg-
ulatory actions that can affect your health.*

49. Rock the Vote

The Ecology of Commerce

By Paul Hawken
Harper Business, 1993, New York.

*Hawken opens your mind to how commerce can reduce pollution and create a
great environment.*

GLOSSARY

Abatement: The act of reducing or making less. Refers to a process in which lead or asbestos levels in a home or building are reduced by a professional contractor.

Acetone: Solvent used in fragrances, drugs, oils, and pesticides. It is an irritant to eyes, skin, lungs, and throat and causes headaches. It can be inhaled or absorbed through the skin.

Acid Rain: Combustion of coal and gasoline emits sulfur into air, combining with moisture to form sulfuric acid and acidified rain. Destroys forests. Kills fish.

Acrylonitrile: Used in making paints, dyes, plastics, synthetic fibers, and pesticides. Causes cancer and nerve damage. Causes headaches, weakness, and skin irritation. Inhaled or absorbed through skin.

Angel dust: See phencyclidine.

Aniline: Used in dyes, inks, resins, varnishes, shoe polishes, drugs, and photo developers. Attacks blood, liver, and heart. Symptoms include: headaches, weakness, irritability, and unconsciousness. Absorbed through skin, eyes, and lungs.

Antioxidants: Certain chemicals change molecules in your body by adding or removing parts and making them unstable. These unstable molecules are called "free radicals" and can cause tissue damage resulting in disease. Antioxidants are minerals and vitamins in foods that have been proven to neutralize these unstable molecules and protect you. Examples of antioxidants are vitamin E, vitamin C, vitamin A, and selenium. Some recent major studies have shown that higher intake of antioxidants is linked with increased life span and decreased risk of disease.

Arsenic: Used in pesticides, enamels, textile printing, drugs, paints, and metal production. Found in drinking water. Attacks skin, eyes, mouth, and throat. Causes cancer. Inhaled or ingested.

Asbestos: Naturally occurring mineral composed of tiny silica fibers. Used in car brakes, insulation, roof coatings, floor and ceiling tiles, and paints. Found in drinking water drawn from rivers that pass over asbestos riverbeds. Lodges in the lungs and causes cancer. Found in homes or buildings, asbestos must be removed under strict safety guidelines.

Aspartame: Artificial sweetener sold under the trade names Nutrasweet and Equal. Made from two amino acids, aspartic acid and phenylalanine, combined with methanol. Linked to brain damage in laboratory animals.

Aspartate: *see* aspartic acid.

Aspartic acid: Amino acid which in high doses acts as excitotoxin in brain. Forty percent of aspartame consumed turns into aspartic acid.

Autism: Condition characterized by disassociation from external reality. Physicians suspect some children diagnosed as autistic suffer from effects of toxins in diet and environment.

Benomyl: Found in fungicides used to wax fruits and vegetables. Associated with birth defects.

Benzene: Found in motor fuels, solvents, inks, paints, plastics, and rubber. Used in making detergents, explosives, drugs, and dyes. Causes cancer and damages nervous system and brain. Inhaled and absorbed through skin and eyes.

Bioaccumulation: Process in which a substance builds up in the body faster than the body can eliminate it.

Blood-brain barrier: Barrier around brain that prevents certain chemicals from entering. Prevents accumulation of toxins and amino acids that cause brain damage. Not fully formed in the unborn or young children. Weakened and penetrated in people who have high blood pressure, diabetes, or cardiovascular disease, or who take psychiatric drugs.

Butyl cellosolve: Derived from oil and widely used in industry and household cleaning products, butyl cellosolve is rapidly absorbed through the skin. It is a nervous system toxin.

Cadmium: Heavy, toxic metal used in metal coatings, solder, nickel plating, jewelry, and catalytic converters in vehicles. Used in fertilizers. Crops grown in these fertilizers, such as tobacco, are high in cadmium. Smokers have high levels of cadmium. Attacks liver, lungs, kidney, and blood. Causes cancer.

Carbaryl: Made from di-isocyanate, the chemical that maimed and killed tens of thousands of people in Bhopal, India, in 1989, carbaryl causes birth defects in dogs and nervous system damage in people.

Carbon dioxide: Colorless, odorless gas emitted from lungs during breathing. Emitted when coal, gasoline, paper, oil, forests burn. Too much carbon dioxide can cause suffocation due to lack of oxygen.

Carbon monoxide: Colorless, odorless, poisonous gas formed by incomplete burning of coal, oil, wood, and gas. Increased reports of carbon monoxide poisoning in homes associated with faulty heaters and ventilation. Gasoline engines emit large amounts.

Carcinogen: A substance that causes cancer in two different species of animals or in humans.

Chelation: From Greek word, *chele,* to claw. Medical treatment giving chemical orally or intravenously to grab or claw heavy metals dissolved in blood and make them insoluble so they pass out of the body through urine. Not effective in removing oil-based toxins from body.

Chlordane: Oil-based pesticide used in United States to kill termites. National Academy of Sciences finds no safe level. Banned in United States in 1980s. Most Americans have accumulated some in their bodies.

Chlorine: Toxic gas used in making bleaches, solvents, pesticides, plastics, and disinfectants. Chlorine in drinking water linked to cancer. Attacks lungs. Inhaled or ingested.

Cobalt: Metal used in pigments, pottery, photographic solutions, and metal plating. Found in drinking water. Irritant to the skin, eyes, and lungs. Linked to heart problems. Inhaled or ingested.

Consumer Product Safety Commission (CPSC): A federal

agency that is responsible for the safety of a wide range of consumer products, other than cosmetics and drugs.

Crystalline silica: A naturally occurring mineral used in a wide range of household and cosmetic products. It is a known human carcinogen.

Cyanuric acid: Chemical used in bleaches. Used in pools to make chlorine last longer (stabilizer) and kill bacteria. Linked to health risks to children at amounts found in pools. Absorbed through skin and lungs and ingested.

DDT: Dichlordiphenyltrichloroethane. Pesticide used throughout world to kill insects. Used on food, as mosquito fogger, and in homes until 1972 when banned in the United States. Causes cancer. Accumulates in human tissue. Americans show DDT in bodies twenty years after ban. Still used in other countries. Can contaminate imported foods.

Detoxification: Several uses: 1.) Body naturally detoxifies certain substances and eliminates these as waste. Liver, kidneys, and skin are detoxification organs. 2.) In drug rehabilitation, a period when someone undergoes physical withdrawal from drug. 3.) A structured program for removing stored toxins from the body.

Diazinon: A member of the organophosphate family of pesticides. It causes nerve and reproductive damage.

Dicloran: Fungicide in wax used to coat fruits and vegetables. Not fully studied for cancer or birth defects.

Dieldrin: Organochlorine pesticide used on crops. Very persistent in environment, accumulates in human fat. Causes cancer and is toxic to nervous system. Absorbed through skin and lungs, also ingested.

Dioxin: Highly toxic chemical formed in production of weed killers, incineration of wastes, or when chlorine contacts wood material and heat. Causes cancer and birth defects. Called the most toxic chemical ever made. Builds up in virtually all animal and human tissues. Found in milk cartons, disposable diapers, napkins, coffee filters, and bleached white paper.

Dursban: A brand name for chlorpyrifos, an organophosphate pesticide. This is one of the most commonly used pesticides around the home by professional exterminators.

Dyslexia: Learning disability affecting person's ability to read. Physicians link some cases to chemicals in environment and diet.

Electromagnetic fields (EMFs): Magnetic fields given off by electrical devices; linked to health problems.

Electromagnetic radiation: Energy with electric and magnetic qualities. X-rays and nuclear radiation are dangerous forms. Light and radio waves are safe forms.

Electrostatic: Term describing electric charges that don't move and attract particles, such as static electricity on sweaters. An electrostatic air filter is good for trapping dust particles.

Environmental Protection Agency: A federal agency given responsibility for protection of humans and the environment.

Ethylbenzene: Contained in gasoline, pesticides, paints, and used in making styrene and synthetic rubber. Primary human exposure from vehicle exhaust (smog) and handling gasoline products. Causes diseases of liver, lungs, kidneys, skin, and lungs. Symptoms include headaches and dizziness. Absorbed through eyes, skin, and lungs.

Ethylene dibromide: Used in pest control and as gasoline additive. Primary human exposure from vehicle exhaust, gasoline evaporation in garages, gasoline pumps, and pesticide fumigation. Causes cancer. Attacks nervous system, lungs, liver, kidneys, and eyes. Inhaled or absorbed through skin and eyes.

Ethylene dichloride: Used in dry cleaning, water softening, glues, cosmetics, drugs, varnishes and as an antiknock agent in gasoline. Causes dizziness and mental confusion. Causes cancer and damages liver, kidneys, and nervous system.

Excitotoxin: Certain essential amino acids, when they reach excessive levels in the body, cease having a beneficial effect and actually overexcite the nervous system, causing cell death. Aspartate in certain artificial sweeteners and glutamate in the food additive monosodium glutamate (MSG) are two such excitotoxins.

Food chain: The natural order of nourishment. Plants grow and are eaten by smaller animals, which are in turn eaten by larger animals, and finally, by man. Toxic chemicals contaminating the chain increase in concentration up to man.

Food and Drug Administration (FDA): A federal agency that, among its many diverse duties, oversees safety issues related to foods, cosmetics, medical drugs for animals and humans, and medical machinery. It is part of the Department of Health and Human Services.

Formaldehyde: Strong-smelling colorless gas used in making particleboard, insulation, and synthetic materials such as carpeting, fibers, and wallpaper. Found in cosmetics as a preservative. Causes cancer and nervous system damage. Inhaled, ingested, or absorbed through eyes and skin.

Free radicals: When a chemical reaction takes place in the body, often caused by environmental toxins, a normally stable molecule becomes unstable and *free* to cause cell and tissue damage.

Fungicides: Synthetic chemicals applied to foods designed to kill fungus, mold, and bacteria.

Gauss unit: Used to measure strength of electromagnetic fields. Named after German scientist Karl Gauss. Health risks are linked to EMFs measured above one one-thousandth of a gauss unit, or 1 milligauss (mG).

General Accounting Office (GAO): A government agency set up to act as a watchdog over other government agencies and issue critical reports, often at the behest of members of Congress. Its reports often reveal facts about government processes and their conflicts of interest that would otherwise remained uncovered.

Glutamate: *See* glutamic acid.

Glutamic acid: Amino acid used in brain to assist nerve function. Comes from diet. Monosodium glutamate and hydrolyzed vegetable protein are major sources. Excess amounts of glutamate in brain are linked to overexcited nerves and brain damage.

Heavy metals: Weight of a metal is determined by its atomic structure—the more atomic particles, the more the weight. Lead, cadmium, mercury, and plutonium are heavy metals, and are toxic.

Herbicide: A type of pesticide designed to eliminate unwanted vegetation.

Hexane: Solvent used to extract oils from foods. Used to decaffeinate coffee and as lab chemical. Nerve toxin. Irritant to skin and eyes. Causes headaches and dizziness. Inhaled, ingested, or absorbed through skin and eyes.

Homeopathy: Alternative medicine, first developed in Europe in the 1800s. Develops medicines for wide variety of illnesses by super-diluting substances that in large doses give same symptoms of the illness. Holistic approach reports significant success.

Hormones: Substances made in the body. Control functions from reproduction to digestion.

Hydrocarbons: Molecules containing hydrogen and carbon, used to produce energy and other chemicals. Benzene is an example. Primary sources of hydrocarbons are crude oil, coal, and natural gas.

Hypersensitive: Condition of reactions and symptoms (headaches, fatigue, nervousness, and depression) to chemicals or foods. Appears to increase if not treated. A number of causes posited, including exposure to toxic chemicals.

Imazalil: Fungicide used in wax coated on fruits and vegetables. Potential ill health effects not completely studied.

Immune system: The natural defense system of the body. Simply, it consists of special white blood cells which attack viruses, bacteria, cancer, and even the common cold. In some diseases the immune system malfunctions and attacks parts of the body, as in diabetes and some forms of arthritis.

Immunotoxic: Term describing toxic chemicals that reduce the body's own defenses against disease.

Indoor pollution: A condition in any building where chemicals from glues, carpets, pesticides, wall coverings, paints, office machinery, tobacco smoke, etc., reach unhealthy levels. The condition is added to by other pollutants such as dust, molds, carbon monoxide and dioxide. It occurs most often when the building lacks adequate ventilation and fresh air.

Ionizing smoke detectors: Use radioactive element to detect presence of smoke.

Kepone: A well-known brand name for chlordecone, a pesticide used on crops to control worms and ants. Causes cancer, infertility, and nerve damage.

Leach: A liquid passing through material brings material with it. Water passing through lead pipes leaches lead. Rainwater passing through a waste dump leaches contaminants.

Lead: Heavy metal used in batteries, pipes, solder, paints, and gasoline manufacture. Primary human exposures: drinking water leached from plumbing; air from vehicle exhausts, smog, and dust from lead-based paints. Accumulates in body, and damages brain and nervous system. Causes lowered IQ, stomach disorders, fatigue, and behavioral problems.

Lesion: Injury or change in tissue or organ resulting in harm or loss of function.

Leukemia: Cancer of the blood and of the organs that manufacture blood cells, principally the bone marrow and lymph nodes and spleen, causing differences in their rate of division, numbers, and function from healthy blood cells. The term "leukemia" comes from the Greek words meaning "white blood," referring to the whitish or pale pink blood in stricken patients. It is the most common childhood cancer.

Lithium: Psychiatric drug often called just a naturally occurring "mineral." It is not. It is a drug, and it has numerous side effects.

Love Canal: Neighborhood in Buffalo, N.Y., where Hooker Chemical dumped toxic wastes into abandoned canal. Homes, schools, and residents were subsequently contaminated with pollutants. Symbolic of public health hazards from toxic waste dumping. Love Canal resident Lois Gibbs was responsible for bringing the issue to public attention.

Lymphoma: A cancer of the lymph glands, one of the most rapidly increasing cancers in the world.

Mercury: Toxic heavy metal used in tooth fillings, metal plating, dyes, leather tanning, felt making, paints, extracting gold and silver, and drugs. Causes irritability, weakness, mouth and gum problems, excitability, anxiety, depression, hallucinations, and muscle tremors. Toxic to nervous system. Stores in body. Inhaled, ingested, or absorbed through eyes and skin.

Methanol: Toxin causing nausea, vomiting, blurred vision, muscular pain, disorientation, weakness, headache, convulsion, and death. Each molecule of aspartame consumed produces one molecule of methanol in blood.

Methyl bromide: Colorless gas or liquid used to treat homes for termites. Residues in carpets, drapes, and leather furniture make people ill. Suspected of causing cancer. Toxic to lungs, skin, and brain.

Methylene chloride: Found in degreasers and paint removers. Narcotic. Causes headache, stupor, irritability, numbness in hands and feet, and irregular heartbeat. Toxic to nervous system. Causes cancer. Inhaled, ingested, or absorbed through skin and eyes.

Monosodium glutamate: Synthetically produced taste enhancer added to food. Produces high levels of glutamate in body; linked to nervous system and brain disorders. An excitotoxin. Contained in food additives not listing it specifically as ingredient.

MSDSs: Manufacturers are required by law to publish the hazards and safety precautions for chemicals used in manufacturing in **M**aterial **S**afety **D**ata **S**heets. These can often provide valuable information to consumers who use products containing these same chemicals.

Nematodes: Microscopic worms occurring naturally in soil, nematodes attack specific pests, but leave other beneficial soil dwellers alone. They do not harm plants, mammals, fish, or birds.

Nervous system: Includes nerves, spinal cord, and brain.

Neurotoxic: Term describing chemicals toxic to nervous system. Cause health problems before cancer. Health effects include lowered IQ, numbness in hands and feet, loss of short-term memory, headache, slower reaction time, loss of concentration, and blurred vision.

Nitrogen oxide: Toxic gas given off by burning natural gas, fuel oil appliances, kerosene heaters, wood burning, and cigarettes. Eye and lung irritant.

Nitrosamines: A family of at least several hundred chemicals, some eighty percent of which cause cancer. Some nitrosamines to which people are commonly exposed are found in consumer products, including household cleaners and cosmetics, as well as cured meats, such as hot dogs. Their presence is the result of a chemical interaction, often between intentionally added ingredients and undisclosed product or food contaminants.

Off-gas: Chemical residues in carpet, wallpaper, glues, paints, cleaners, sprays, dry-cleaned clothes, stains, and waxes that volatilize into air. Contributes to indoor pollution.

Optical smoke detector: Detects smoke visually.

Organochlorines: Group of pesticides and similar substances combining oil-based chemicals with chlorine. Includes DDT, Agent Orange, chlordane, PCBs, and dioxin. Do not break down, and accumulate in environment and food chain. Virtually every American has measurable amounts in fat.

Organophosphates: Group of pesticides made with petroleum chemicals combined with phosphoric acid. Toxic to human nervous system. First developed as chemical warfare agents.

Ortho-phenylphenol: Fungicide used in wax coatings applied to fruits and vegetables. Suppresses immune system. Causes cancer.

Oxidation: A chemical process in which the positive electric charge of an atom or molecule is increased. When this occurs the resulting atom or molecule is typically less stable.

Ozonator: Machine that generates ozone into water to kill bacteria. Used broadly, instead of chlorine, to disinfect water in Europe. Increasingly used in United States to disinfect pool water.

Ozone: Pale blue gas, a form of oxygen with a sharp smell. At ground level is the main component of smog. Some twenty to fifty kilometers above the earth's surface, ultraviolet (UV) radiation splits a molecule of oxygen (O_2) into two reactive atoms. If one of these atoms encounters another oxygen molecule, an ozone molecule (O_3) is formed. The thin layer of ozone in the stratosphere absorbs the sun's ultraviolet radiation, protecting plants and animals from its adverse effects. Closer to the earth, ozone is a powerful lung irritant.

Particleboard: Wood product made from wood chips and formaldehyde-based glue. Used in low-cost furniture, paneling, floor boards, and shelving. Gives off formaldehyde fumes.

PCBs: Polychlorinated biphenyls. Invented in the 1930s and added to oil inside electrical devices to protect oil breakdown at high temperatures. They conduct electricity and resist heat, requiring three thousand degrees to break down. Most PCBs made are still in the environment, despite being banned in the 1970s as toxic and cancer causing. Found in water, soil, fish, crops, animals, and humans today.

Pesticides: Chemicals used to destroy pests, including weeds, rodents, and insects. Sprayed on fruits, grains, and vegetables.

Insecticides and herbicides are under its general heading.

Petrochemicals: Chemicals made from petroleum.

Petroleum: Flammable, oily liquid made up of hydrocarbons found in ground as crude oil.

Phencyclidine: Angel dust. Illegal drug used as dip for cigarettes and marijuana. Causes hallucinations and overexcitement. Law enforcement officers are exposed during raids on illegal labs. Oil-based and stores in human fat. Linked to flashbacks in drug users and exposed police officers.

Phenylalanine: An essential amino acid for normal brain function. In excessive amounts causes brain damage, seizures, hyperactivity, and retardation. Consumption of aspartame with carbohydrates increases phenylalanine levels in body.

4 Phenylcyclohexane (4-PC): Toxic chemical found in latex backing of synthetic carpets. Fumes linked to health complaints including allergies, headaches, fatigue, increased chemical sensitivity, and immune system disorders.

Photoelectric smoke detector: Uses light and an electric charge to detect smoke.

Phytomin: The numerous, many as yet unidentified, disease-preventing substances in whole foods such as fruits and vegetables. Scientists believe these to be a potent new nutritional weapon against disease.

Polyethylene: Plastic used in carpet, chewing gum, coffee stirrers, drinking glasses, food containers, plastic bags, garbage cans, toys, and squeeze bottles. Suspected of causing cancer.

Polyoxyethlene: A toxic chemical added to pools to control algae.

Polystyrene: A plastic used in model kits, floor polishes, ice buckets, and fast-food cups and containers. Styrene can leach from these containers into food and drink and is found in virtually all Americans. A common form, "Styrofoam," is a trade name.

Polyvinyl chloride: Plastic used in artificial grass, baby pants, cosmetics, crib bumpers, floor tiles, pipes, garden hoses, inflatable toys, pacifiers, and shower curtains. Releases vinyl chloride that causes cancer and birth defects.

Press-wood: *See* particleboard.

Prozac: The brand name for Fluoxetine. Psychiatric drug made by

Eli Lilly, tied to numerous reports of violence and suicides. Reported side effects exceed all similar drugs combined.

Radon: Naturally occurring radioactive gas, common to certain rock formations in Midwest and East. Builds up in basements of homes not properly vented. Second leading cause of lung cancer in United States.

Ritalin: Methylphenidate. Addictive, speed-like drug prescribed for hyperactive children. Associated with numerous ill side effects. Wrongly prescribed when environmental toxins are the actual cause of behavioral problems.

Sebum: Oil excreted from human skin.

Sensitizer: A chemical that creates symptoms in certain individuals often at lower doses and before similar symptoms would manifest in others. There are a number of theories concerning this reaction, but reports are that some people sensitized by one chemical become increasingly sensitive to other chemicals in their environments.

Shellac: Thin coating made from alcohol and petroleum resins used in varnishes. Used in coating fruits and vegetables.

Sodium ortho-phenyl phenate: Fungicide used in wax coatings applied to fruits and vegetables. Suspected of causing cancer.

Solvent: Liquid that dissolves or can dissolve another substance. Water is a solvent for table salt. Cleaners, degreasers, oven cleaners, car cleaners, dry cleaning fluids, spot removers, and paint thinners are solvents. Most industrial solvents are made from petroleum.

Styrene: Used in production of plastics and drugs. Suspected of causing cancer and ailments including dizziness, fatigue, nervousness, difficulty sleeping, poor memory, and skin and lung irritation. Stored in human tissue.

Synergy and synergism: The often unpredictable interactions of chemical substances, such as contaminants or drugs, that, when combined, enhance each other's effectiveness.

THC: Tetrahydrocannabinol. Psychoactive ingredient in marijuana. Linked to brain damage, reduced fertility, and lung disease. Stores in body. Far deadlier than first thought. Concentration in marijuana in 1960s was one percent; today, twelve percent. Irreparable damage linked to concentrations over four percent.

Toluene: Solvent used in production of chemicals, found in vehicle fuels and paints. Causes headache, fatigue, weakness, staggering, and skin irritation. Toxic to nervous system. Inhaled and absorbed through skin.

Toxicology: The study of poisons, their effects, and cures.

Toxin: Poisonous substance, whether in solid, liquid, or gas form. It harms life.

Trichloroethane: Methyl chloroform. Solvent used for degreasing and cleaning. Used as dry-cleaning chemical and propellant. Causes dizziness, reduced reaction time, and lack of coordination. Toxic to nervous system. Inhaled, ingested, or absorbed through eyes and skin.

Trichloroethylene: Solvent used in degreasing, dry cleaning, decaffeinating coffee, and production of pesticides, waxes, and paints. Found in drinking water. Causes headache, fatigue, blurred vision, and irregular heart beat. Causes cancer. Toxic to nervous system. Inhaled, ingested, and absorbed through skin.

2,4-D: A widely used herbicide available at most garden shops, it is associated with cancer among farmers who use it in the Midwest and Corn Belt. It used to be one-half of the formulation called Agent Orange used to destroy the jungles of Vietnam.

Ultraviolet: Form of electromagnetic radiation with a wavelength shorter than violet light. Used to kill bacteria in water.

U.S.D.A.: United States Department of Agriculture.

Valium: Diazepam. Highly addictive tranquilizer. Stores in body.

Vinyl chloride: Toxic gas used in production of polyvinyl chloride plastics. (See polyvinyl chloride.) Causes cancer. Toxic to nervous system. Inhaled.

Xanax: A brand name for the anti-depressant drug alprazolam. This drug can cause birth defects if taken by a pregnant woman. People using this drug are advised not to drive or perform any task that requires mental alertness. Common side effects include drowsiness, depression, headache, and nervousness.

Xenoestrogen: As their name implies, xenoestrogens are not natural estrogens. They are produced outside of the human body, but scientists have discovered that once they find their way into the human body a number of these structurally disparate petrochemicals, including a wide range of pesticides and industrial pollutants, have the uncanny ability to mimic estrogen, the primary feminizing hormone; they evoke "responses in the uterus [or other female reproductive organs] similar to those observed after administration of classical estrogens, such as estradiol." Other demonstrable effects in both experimental animals and wildlife include stimulating cell proliferation in reproductive organs and abnormal enlargement of secondary female sexual organs.

Xylene: Solvent chemical found in paints, glues, dyes, varnishes, cleaning fluids, and aviation fuels. Irritant to eyes, skin, and lungs. Depresses nervous system. Attacks kidneys and liver. Inhaled, ingested, and absorbed through eyes and skin.

NOTES

4. Clean House

1. Sterling, D.A. Presentation at National Center for Health Statistics Conference. Washington, D.C., July 15, 17, 1991.
2. International Agency for Research on Cancer, supplement 7, 1987, pp. 341–342.
3. Consumer Product Safety Commission. "Product summary report." National Electronic Injury Surveillance System. National Injury Information Clearinghouse, Washington, D.C., 1990.
4. See note 1 above.
5. See note 1 above.
6. Steinman, D. & Epstein, S.S. *The Safe Shopper's Bible*. New York: Macmillan, 1995, pp. 1–28.
7. *Occupational Exposure to Ethylene Glycol Monobutyl Ether and Ethylene Glycol Monobutyl Ether Acetate*. Cincinnati, Ohio: National Institute for Occupational Safety and Health, September 1990.
8. Vincent, R., et al. *Applied Industrial Hygiene,* June 1993.
9. Steinman & Epstein. *The Safe Shopper's Bible,* pp. 71–72.
10. Material Safety Data Sheets (MSDS) October 3, 1988; January 6, 1989; June 20, 1990; March 13, 1991; August 13, 1991; January 6, 1992; April 22, 1992.
11. Hill, R. H., et al. "p-Dichlorobenzene exposure among 1000 adults in the United States." *Archives of Environmental Health,* 1995. 50(4): 277–280.
12. Guy, R. & Potts, R. *American Journal of Industrial Medicine,* May 1993.
13. Dadd, D. "Cleaning products," *The Nontoxic Home and Office.* Los Angeles: Jeremy Tarcher, Inc., 1992, p. 11.
14. Dadd, D. *The Nontoxic Home.* Los Angeles: Jeremy Tarcher, Inc., 1986, p. 10.
15. Sanders, B. "News and Updates." *Greenkeeping: The Environmental Consumer's Guide,* Vol. 2 No. 2, Lebanon, N.H., May/June 1992, p. 3.
16. Sittig, M. *Handbook of Toxic and Hazardous Chemicals and Carcinogens,* Second Edition, Park Ridge, N.J.: Noyes Publications, 1985, p. 652.
17. Ibid., pp. 71, 217, 261, 462, 695, 704.
18. Ibid., pp. 71, 718, 815.

200   *Notes*

19. Ibid., p. 313.
20. Ibid., pp. 71, 718, 815.

5. Pull the Rug Out

1. Anderson, R. L. "Biological evaluation of carpeting." *Applied Microbiology,* 1969, pp. 180–187.
2. Hirzy, W. & Morison, R. "Carpet/4-phenylcyclohexane toxicity: the EPA headquarters case." Washington, D.C.: National Federation of Federal Employees, 1989.
3. Sittig, M. *Handbook of Toxic and Hazardous Chemicals and Carcinogens,* Second Edition, Park Ridge, N.J.: Noyes Publications, 1985, p. 528.
4. Ibid., p. 805.
5. Zamm, A. *Why Your House May Endanger Your Health.* New York: Simon & Schuster, 1980, p. 98.
6. Brower, N. *The Healthy Household.* Bloomington, Ind.: The Healthy House Institute, 1995, pp. 118–119.
7. Beebe, G. *Toxic Carpet III:* "Consumer product complaint reports." Cincinnati, Ohio: Beebe, 1991, pp. 252–323.
8. Anonymous. "ARN tests 'low allergy' vacuum cleaners." *Rodale's Allergy Relief,* 1987, 2(11).
9. Patriarca, P. "Kawasaki syndrome: association with the application of rug shampoo." *The Lancet,* 1982: 578–580.
10. Monsanto Corporation. "Carpet emissions test requirements." Memorandum, 1990.

6. What's That Dirty, Gauzy Thing in My Furnace?

1. Oge, M. & Farland, W. "Radon risk in the home." *Science,* 1992, 255: 1194–1195.
2. Mott, L. & Snyder, K. *Pesticide Alert: A Guide to Pesticides in Fruits and Vegetables.* San Francisco: Sierra Club Books, 1987.
3. National Research Council. *Pesticides in the Diets of Infants and Children.* Washington, D.C.: National Academy Press, 1993.
4. Sittig, M. *Handbook of Toxic and Hazardous Chemicals and Carcinogens,* Second Edition, Park Ridge, N.J.: Noyes Publications, 1985.
5. Browner, C. "Environmental tobacco smoke: EPA's report." *EPA Journal,* Washington, D.C.: Environmental Protection Agency, 1993, 19(4): 13.
6. Pope, A. "Indoor allergens report." *EPA Journal,* Washington, D.C.: Environmental Protection Agency, 1993, 19(4): 19.
7. Haymore, C. & Odom, R. "Economic effects of poor indoor air quality." *EPA Journal.* Washington, D.C.: Environmental Protection Agency, 1993, 28–29.

7. Paint Your Wagon

1. Curtis, D.L., et al. "Interim report on medical testing protocol: Los Angeles County Painters Trust." Los Angeles, 1986.

2. Selinger, B. *Chemistry in the Marketplace.* Canberra, Australia: Australian National University Press, 1981, p. 182.

3. Sittig, M. *Handbook of Toxic and Hazardous Chemicals and Carcinogens.* Park Ridge, N.J.: Noyes Publications, 1986.

4. Flick, E. *Handbook of Paint Raw Materials.* Park Ridge, N.J.: Noyes Publications, 1982, pp. 1–2.

5. Gooselin, R., et al. *Clinical Toxicology of Commercial Products.* Baltimore: Williams and Watkins, 1984, pp. 2–84.

6. Monster, A. "Biological markers of solvent exposure." *Archives of Environmental Health,* 1988, 43(2): 90–92.

7. United States Environmental Protection Agency. *Broad Scan Analysis of the FY82 National Human Adipose Tissue Survey Specimens: Volume I—Executive Summary.* Washington, D.C.: 1986, EPA-560/5-86-035.

8. van Faassen, A. & Borm, P. "Composition and health hazards of water-based construction paints: results from a survey in the Netherlands." *Environmental Health Perspectives,* 1991, 92: 147–154.

9. *International Agency For Research On Cancer Monographs on the Evaluation of Carcinogen Risks to Humans. Some organic solvents, resin monomers and related compounds, pigments and occupational exposures in paint manufacture and painting.* Lyon, France: World Health Organization, 1989, 47: 422–447.

10. Ibid.

11. Chisolm, J.J. & Farfel, R. The Kennedy Institute for Handicapped Children.

8. Wired!

1. Brodeur, P., *The Great Power Line Cover-Up.* Boston: Little, Brown and Company, 1993.

2. Wertheimer, N. & Leeper, E. "Electrical wiring configurations and childhood cancer." *American Journal of Epidemiology,* 1979, 109: 273–284.

3. Wertheimer, N. & Leeper, E. "Adult cancer related to electric wires near the home." *International Journal of Epidemiology,* 1982, 11: 345–355.

4. Ketchen, E., et al. "The biological effects of magnetic fields on man." *American Industrial Hygiene Association Journal,* 1978, 39: 1–11.

5. Brower, N. *The Healthy Household.* Bloomington, Ind.: The Healthy House Institute, 1995, pp. 379–391.

6. Ibid.

7. Breysse, P. "ELF magnetic field exposures in an office environment." *American Journal of Industrial Medicine,* 1994, 25: 177–185.

8. Brodeur, P. *The Great Power Line Cover-Up,* pp. 66, 75, 134, 181, 273–274.

9. Ibid., pp. 49–50.

10. Ibid., p. 83.

11. Ibid., p. 47.

12. Brower, N. *The Healthy Household,* p. 385.

13. Brodeur, P. *The Great Power Line Cover-Up,* p. 254.

9. Are You Glowing in the Dark?

1. Stammer, L. "Test homes for radon, EPA says." *Los Angeles Times,* September 13, 1988.

2. Ibid.

3. Anonymous. "More risks seen in low-level radiation." *The Nation's Health.* Washington, D.C.: The American Public Health Association, 1990.

4. Kashdan, E., et al. "Review of recent research in indoor air quality." Washington, D.C.: Environmental Protection Agency, 1984, EPA-600/2-84-009.

5. Chessin, R., et al. "Update of indoor air quality bibliography." Triangle Park, N.C.: Research Triangle Institute, 1992, RTI/3065/05-03F, 68-02-3992-005.

6. *Bibliography on Indoor Air Pollution,* Washington, D.C.: Environmental Protection Agency, 1985, EPA/IMSD-85-002.

7. Darby, S., et al. "Radon and cancers other than lung cancer in underground miners: a collaborative analysis of 11 studies." *Journal of the National Cancer Institute,* 1995, 87(5): 378–384.

8. Darling, J., et al. "Lung cancer in radon-exposed miners and estimation of risk from indoor exposure. *Journal of the National Cancer Institute,* 1995, 87(11): 817–827.

9. See note 1 above.

10. Freeze 'Em, Zap 'Em

1. Sherman, J.D. *Chemical Exposure and Disease.* Princeton, N.J.: Princeton Scientific Publishing Co., Inc., 1994, p. 138.

2. Epstein, S.S. "Corporate crime: why we cannot trust industry-derived safety studies." *International Journal of Health Services,* 1990, 20(3): 443–458.

3. Ibid.

4. Sherman, J.D. *Chemical Exposure and Disease,* pp. 144–145.

5. Gips, T. *Breaking the Pesticide Habit.* Penang, Malaysia: International Organization of Consumers Unions, 1987, pp. 92–108.

6. *International Agency for Research on Cancer (IARC) Monographs,* 1979, 20: 45–65, 129–154.

7. Blair, A., et al. "Lung cancer and other causes of death among licensed pesticide applicators." *Journal of the National Cancer Institute,* 1983, 71: 31–37.

8. Ditraglia, D., et al. "Mortality study of workers employed at organochlorine pesticide manufacturing plants." *Scandinavian Journal of Work, Environment and Health,* 1981, 7 (supplement 4): 1401–46.

9. Wang, H.H. & MacMahon, B. "Mortality of workers employed in the manufacture of chlordane and heptachlor." *Journal of Occupational Medicine,* 1979, 21: 745–748.

10. Sherman, J.D. *Chemical Exposure and Disease,* p. 147.

11. *IARC Monographs,* 1987, 41: 187–212.

12. Ibid.

13. Boorman, G.A., et al. "Regression of methyl bromide-induced forestomach lesions in the rat." *Toxicology and Applied Pharmacology,* 1986, 86: 131–139.

14. Briggs, S.A. & Rachel Carson Council. *Basic Guide to Pesticides: Their Characteristics and Hazards.* Washington, D.C.: Taylor & Francis, 1992, p. 164.

15. Ibid., p. 186.

16. Ibid., p. 115.

17. Sherman, J.D. *Chemical Exposure and Disease.* pp. 144–145.

18. See note 16 above.

19. United States Environmental Protection Agency. "Registration standard (second round review) for the reregistration of pesticide products containing chlorpyrifos." June 1989, p. 42.

20. Burin, G.J. Memorandum to Ellenberger, J. "Chlorpyrifos registration standard." Environmental Protection Agency, Office of Pesticides and Toxic Substances, May 25, 1984.

21. Fenske, R.A., et al. "Potential exposure and health risks of infants following indoor residential pesticide applications." *American Journal of Public Health,* 1990, 80(6): 689–693.

22. Sherman, J.D. *Chemical Exposure and Disease.* pp. 140–141.

23. Metcalf, R. *Introduction to Integrated Pest Management,* 2nd ed., New York: Wiley, 1982, p. 294.

24. "Natural pesticides from the neem tree and other tropical plants." *Proceedings of the Second International Neem Conference,* Rauschholzhausen, Federal Republic of Germany, May 25–28, 1983, Eschborn, FRG: GTZ, 1985.

25. Hansen, M. *Pest Control for Home and Garden,* Yonkers, N.Y.: Consumers Union, 1993, pp. 136–142.

26. Ibid.

27. See note 5 above.

11. I Promise You a Rose Garden

1. Ellis, B.W. & Bradley, F.M., editors. *The Organic Gardener's Handbook of Natural Insect and Disease Control.* Emmaus, Pa.: Rodale Press, 1992, p. 258.

2. Lowengart, R.A., et al. "Childhood leukemia and parent's occupational and home exposures." *Journal of the National Cancer Institute,* 1987, 79: 39–46.

3. Davis, J.R., et al. "Family pesticide use and childhood brain cancer." *Archives of Environmental Contamination and Toxicology,* 1993, 24: 87–92.

4. Richardson, S., et al. "Occupational risk factors for acute leukemia: a case-control study." *International Journal of Epidemiology,* 1992, 21(6): 1063–1073.

5. National Coalition Against the Misuse of Pesticides (NCAMP). Statement of Jay Feldman, national coordinator, before the Subcommittee on Toxic Substances, Environmental Oversight, Research and Development Committee on Environment and Public Works, U.S. Senate, May 9, 1991.

6. Ellis & Bradley, *The Organic Gardener's Handbook,* p. 462.

7. Cherim, M. *Green Methods Catalog.* Barrington, N.H.: Department of Bio-Ingenuity, 1995, p. 18.

8. Ellis & Bradley, *The Organic Gardener's Handbook,* p. 454.

9. Ibid.

10. Ibid.

11. Ibid.

12. Ibid., p. 456.
13. Ibid.
14. Ibid.
15. *Natural Products for Lawn, Garden & Farm.* Bozeman, Mont.: Bozeman Bio-Tech. Not dated, p. 15.
16. Ibid.
17. Ibid.
18. Ellis & Bradley, *The Organic Gardener's Handbook,* p. 485.
19. Ibid.
20. Ibid.

12. My Life as a Dog

1. National Research Council. *Animals as Sentinels of Environmental Health Hazards.* Committee on Animals as Monitors of Environmental Hazards, Board of Environmental Studies and Toxicology, Commission on Life Sciences, Natural Research Council. Washington, D.C.: National Academy Press, 1991, pp. 72–73.
2. Graham, E. "Fleas start to yield their blood secrets to dogged research." *The Wall Street Journal,* December 28, 1993, A1–A2.
3. Engler, R. "List of chemicals evaluated for carcinogenic potential." Memorandum. United States Environmental Protection Agency, Health Effects Division, October 14, 1992, p. 3.
4. Briggs, S.A. & Rachel Carson Council. *Basic Guide to Pesticides. Their Characteristics and Hazards.* Washington, D.C.: Taylor & Francis, 1992: 158.
5. Engler. "List of chemicals," p. 5
6. Briggs & Carson Council. *Basic Guide to Pesticides,* p. 177.
7. Ibid., p. 181.
8. Ibid., p. 183.
9. Hansen, M. *Pest Control for Home and Garden.* Yonkers, N.Y.: Consumers Union, 1993, p. 293.
10. Ibid., p. 210.
11. Steinman, D. & Epstein, S.S. *The Safe Shopper's Bible.* New York: Macmillan, 1995, pp. 122–133.
12. See note 1 above.
13. Davis, J.R., et al. "Family pesticide use and childhood brain cancer." *Archives of Environmental Contamination and Toxicology,* 1993, 24: 87–92.
14. Ames, R.G., et al. "Health symptoms and occupational exposure to flea control products among California pet handlers." *Journal of the American Industrial Hygiene Association,* 1989, 50(9): 466–472.
15. Ibid.
16. Anonymous. "Guide to a pest-free pet." *Consumer Reports,* August 1991, p. 563.
17. Briggs & Carson Council. *Basic Guide to Pesticides,* p. 211.
18. Ibid., p. 158.
19. See note 14 above.
20. Steinman, D. & Dodds, J. "Are you loving your pet to death?" *Safe & Healthy,* 1995.
21. Material Safety Data Sheet, FleaBusters, Ft. Lauderdale, Fla., March 21, 1991.

22. Brennan, M.L. & Eckroate, N. *The Natural Dog.* New York: Plume, 1994, p. 261.
23. Hansen, M. *Pest Control for Home and Garden,* pp. 210–211.
24. Scarff, D.H. & Lloyd, D.H. "Double blind, placebo-controlled, crossover study of evening primrose oil in the treatment of canine atopy." *The Veterinary Record,* pp. 97–99, August 1, 1992.
25. Brennan & Eckroate. *The Natural Dog,* pp. 262–263.
26. Ibid.
27. Ibid., p. 264.

13. Attack of the Killer House . . . Building It Better

1. Surman, B. "Worst pollutants found indoors, scientists say." *Los Angeles Times,* September 11, 1986, p. 26.
2. Carey, J., Hager, M., King, P., Zuckerman, S. "Beware 'sick-building syndrome.'" *Newsweek: Health,* January 7, 1985, p. 58.
3. Ossler, C. "Men's work environment and health risks." *Nursing Clinics of North America,* March, 1986, 21: 25–36.
4. "Dust to dust." *USA Today,* October 28, 1986, p. D1.
5. "Indoor smog." *Newsweek,* May 30, 1977, p. 78.
6. Zamm, A. & Gannon, R. *Why Your House May Endanger Your Health.* New York: Simon & Schuster, 1982, pp. 131–132.
7. Rylander, R., et al. *Scandinavian Journal of Work, Environment and Health,* 1991.
8. Gunby, P. "Fact or fiction about formaldehyde." *Journal of the American Medical Association,* 1980, 243: 1697.
9. "Formaldehyde: evidence of carcinogencity." *Current Intelligence Bulletin 34.* Cincinnati, Ohio: National Institute for Occupational Safety and Health, 1981, DHHS (NIOSH) #81–111.
10. Ritchie, I. & Lehnen, R. "Formaldehyde-related health complaints of residents living in mobile and conventional homes." *American Journal of Public Health,* 1987, 77(3): 323–327.
11. Kilburn, K. & Warshaw, R. "Formaldehyde impairs memory, equilibrium, and dexterity in histology technicians: effects which persist for days." *Archives of Environmental Health,* 1987, 42(2): 117–120.
12. Rousseau, D., Rea, W., Enwright, J. *Your Home, Your Health & Your Well-Being.* Berkeley, Cal.: Ten Speed Press, 1988.
13. Bergin, E. & Grandon, R. *How to Survive in Your Toxic Environment.* New York: Avon Books, 1984, p. xiv.

15. Honey, There's a Monster in the Pool!

1. Bergin, E. & Grandon, R. *How to Survive in Your Toxic Environment.* New York: Avon Books, 1984, pp. 24–26.
2. Shaffer, M. "Chlorine may spur swimmers' asthma." *Medical Tribune,* July 24, 1992, p. 34.
3. See note 1 above.

4. Milunsky, A. "Maternal heat exposure and neural tube defects." *Journal of the American Medical Association,* 1992, 268(7): 882–885.

16. Just Say No!

1. Hart, R. *Pot in a Nutshell.* Topsfield, Mass.: Committees of Correspondence, 1986, p. 1.
2. Anonymous. "Fate and distribution of cocaine, diazepam, phencyclidine and THC (marijuana): a technical review." Los Angeles: Foundation for Advancements in Science and Education, 1985, 1–4.
3. Friedman, H., et al. "Tissue distribution of diazepam and its metabolite desmethyldiazepam: a human autopsy study." *Journal of Clinical Pharmacology,* 1985, 25: 613–615.
4. Nayak, M., et al. "Physiological disposition and biotransformation of cocaine in acutely and chronically treated rats." *The Journal of Pharmacology and Experimental Therapeutics,* 1974, 196: 556–569.
5. Stolman, A. *Progress in Chemical Toxicology: Volume 5.* New York: Academic Press, 1974, pp. 1–99.
6. See note 2 above.
7. Peterson, R. "Marijuana health report." Report to U.S. Congress. Washington, D.C., 1980: 3.
8. Nahas, G. "Pharmacological and epidemiological aspects of alcohol and cannabis." *New York State Journal of Medicine,* 1984, 84: 82–87.
9. Crow, T.J., et al. "Two syndromes in schizophrenia and their pathogenesis." *Schizophrenia as a Brain Disease.* New York: Oxford University Press, 1982, p. 204.
10. Tashkin, D.P. "Subacute effects of heavy marijuana smoking on pulmonary function in healthy men." *New England Journal of Medicine,* 1988, 294(3): 125–129.
11. Oliwenstein, L., "The perils of pot." *Discover,* June 1988, 18.
12. Ricaurte, G., et al. "Hallucinogenic amphetamine selectively destroys brain serotonin terminals." *Science,* 1985, 229: 986–988.
13. Rothlin, E., et al. "Preliminary studies of the metabolism of lysergic acid and diethylamide using radioactive carbon-marked molecules." *Journal of Pharmacology and Experimental Therapy,* 1955, 113: 6.
14. Farrow, J. & Van Vunakis. "Binding of *d*-lysergic acid diethylamide to subcellular fractions from rat brain." *Nature,* 1972, 237: 164–165.
15. Boyd, E., et al. "Preliminary studies of the metabolism of lysergic acid diethylamide using radioactive carbon-marked molecules." *Journal of Mental and Nervous Disorders,* 1955, 122: 470–471.
16. Cone, E. & Weddington, W. "Prolonged occurrence of cocaine in human saliva and urine after chronic use." *Journal of Analytical Toxicology,* 1989, 13: 65–68.
17. Weiss, R. "Protracted elimination of cocaine metabolites in long-term, high-dose cocaine abusers." *American Journal of Medicine,* 1988, 85: 879–880.
18. See note 3 above.
19. Martin, B. "Long-term disposition of phencyclidine in mice." *Drug Metabolism and Distribution,* 1982, 10(2): 189–193.
20. James, S. & Schnoll, S. "Phencyclidine: tissue distribution in the rat." *Clinical Toxicology,* 1976, 9: 573–582.

21. Laposata, E. & Lange, L. "Presence of nonoxidative ethanol metabolism in human organs commonly damaged by ethanol abuse." *Science,* 1986, 231: 497–499.

22. Horstman, D., et al. "Lipid metabolism during heavy and moderate exercise." *Journal of Sports Medicine,* 1971, 3: 18–23.

23. Smart, R.G. & Bateman, K. "Review article: unfavorable reactions to LSD: a review and analysis of the available case reports." *Journal of Canadian Medical Association,* 1967, 97: 1214–1221.

24. Harmer, R. *American Medical Avarice.* New York: Abelard & Schulman, 1975, p. 183.

25. Loomis, D. "Which is safer: drugs or vitamins?" *American Journal of Emergency Medicine,* 1992, 105: 219.

26. Anonymous. "Drug money and data fudging." *Townsend Letter for Doctors,* November 1994, 1167.

27. Rochon, P., et al. "A study of manufacturer-supported trials of nonsteroidal anti-inflammatory drugs in the treatment of arthritis." *Archives of Internal Medicine,* 1994, 154: 157–163.

28. See note 24 above.

29. Marx, J. "Do anti-depressants promote tumors?" *Science,* 1992, 257: 22–23.

30. Anonymous. "Drugs that cause sexual dysfunction: an update." *The Medical Letter,* 1992, 34(876): 73–78

31. Shields, M.D.G. "Reassessing Prozac." *Newsweek,* April 1, 1991.

32. FDA Spontaneous Reporting System. Washington, D.C.: Food and Drug Administration, 1991.

17. What's Up, Doc?

1. National Research Council. *The Role of the Primary Care Physician in Occupational and Environmental Medicine.* Washington, D.C.: Institute of Medicine, National Academy Press, 1988.

2. Ibid.

3. Bergin, E. & Grandon, R. *How to Survive in Your Toxic Environment.* New York: Avon Books, 1984, p. 165.

4. Boyle, R. & Environmental Defense Fund. *Malignant Neglect.* New York: Alfred Knopf, 1979, pp. 206–207.

5. Harris, S. & Highland, J. "Birthright denied." Washington, D.C.: Environmental Defense Fund, 1977, p. 11.

18. A Phytomin a Day Keeps the Toxins Away

1. Byers, T. & Perry, G. "Dietary carotenes, vitamin C, and vitamin E as protective antioxidants in human cancers." *Annual Review of Nutrition,* 1992, 12: 139–159.

2. Greenwald, P. "Experience from clinical trials in cancer prevention." *Annals of Medicine,* 1994, 26: 73–80.

3. See note 1 above.

4. Mullaart, E., et al. "DNA damage metabolism and aging." *Mutation Research* 237; 1990: 189–210.

5. Mohsen, M. "Impact of aging on detoxification mechanisms." *Nutritional Toxicology.* New York: Mackey, Maureen, Raven Press, Ltd., chapter Ili: 49–66.

6. Ibid.

7. Hudecova, A. & Ginter, E. "The influence of ascorbic acid on lipid peroxidation in guinea pigs intoxicated with cadmium." *Federation of Chemical Toxicology,* 1992, 30(12): 1011–1013.

8. Amagase, H., et al. "Garlic helps inhibit cancer." *The Nutrition Report,* January 1994, 3.

9. Amagase, H. & Milner, J.A. "Impact of various sources of garlic and their constituents on 7,12-dimethylbenz[a]anthracene binding to mammary cell DNA." *Carcinogenesis,* August 1993, 14(8): 1627–1631.

10. Reiter, R.J. "Pineal gland, cellular proliferation and neoplastic growth: an historical account." *The Pineal Gland and Cancer.* [eds. Gupta, D., et al.]. Brain Research Promotion, Tübingen, Germany, 1988, 41–64.

11. Gao, Y.T., et al. "Reduced risk of esophageal cancer associated with green tea consumption." *Journal of the National Cancer Institute,* 1994, 86: 855–858.

12. Mukhtar, H., et al. "Tea components: antimutagenic and anticarcinogenic effects." *Preventive Medicine,* 1992, 21: 351–360.

19. Get Smart!

1. Florini, K. & Silbergeld, E. "Getting the lead out." *Issues in Science and Technology,* 1993, 4: 33–39.

2. Bellinger, D. "Low level lead exposure and children's cognitive function in preschool years." *Pediatrician,* 1991, 87(2): 219–227.

3. Kilburn, K. "Is the nervous system most sensitive to environmental toxins?" *Archives of Environmental Health,* 1989, 44(6): 343–344.

4. Sciarillo, W., et al. "Lead exposure and child behavior." *American Journal of Public Health,* 1992, 82(10): 1356–1357.

5. Wacker, J. "Learning disabilities: diet and chemical exposure." *Latitudes,* 1994, 1(3–4): 3.

6. See note 1 above.

7. Blaylock, R. *Excitotoxins: The Taste That Kills.* Santa Fe, N.M.: Health Press, 1995.

8. Brostoff, J. & Gamlin, L. *Food Allergy and Intolerance.* London: Bloomsbury Publishing Limited, 1989.

9. Rapp, D. *Is This Your Child?* New York: William Morrow and Company, 1991.

10. Connors, C., et al. "Food additives and hyperkinesis: a controlled double-blind experiment." *Pediatrics,* 1976, (58): 154.

11. Wisner, R. & Shields, G. "Treatment of children with the detoxification method developed by Hubbard." Annual Meeting of American Academy of Environmental Medicine, 1992.

12. Damstra, T. & McMahon, A. "Tots & toxins: altered brains." *Latitudes,* 1994, 1(3–4): 7.

13. Natural Resources Defense Council. *Twenty-Five-Year Report* (1970–1995). New York: Natural Resources Defense Council, 1995, p. 14.

14. Florini & Silbergeld. "Getting the lead out," p. 35.

15. National Research Council. *Pesticides in the Diets of Infants and Children.* Washington, D.C.: National Academy Press, 1993, p. 3.

16. Swell, B. & Whyatt, R. "Intolerable risks: pesticides in our children's food." New York: Natural Resources Defense Council, 1989.

17. Buttram, H. *Volatile Organic Compounds: Contributory Causes of Learning Disabilities and Behavioral Problems in Children.* Blooming Glen, Pa.

20. Don't Sweat It . . . Yes, Do!

1. Elkington, J. *The Poisoned Womb.* New York: Penguin Books, 1985, pp. 235–236.

2. Council on Environmental Quality. *The Sixth Annual Report of the Council on Environmental Quality,* Washington, D.C.: Council on Environmental Quality, 1975, p. 369.

3. Environmental Protection Agency. *Broad Scan Analysis of the FY82 National Human Adipose Tissue Survey Specimens: Volume I—Executive Summary.* Washington, D.C.: Environmental Protection Agency, 1986, EPA-560/5-86-035.

4. Carson, R. *Silent Spring.* Boston: Houghton Mifflin Company, 1962.

5. Weilbacher, M. "Toxic shock: the environment-cancer connection." *E The Environmental Magazine,* 1995, 6(3): 30.

6. Wolff, M.S., et al. "Human tissue burdens of halogenated aromatic chemicals in Michigan." *Journal of the American Medical Association,* 1982, 247: 2112–2116.

7. Vree, T., et al. "Excretion of amphetamines in human sweat." *Archives Internal Pharmacodynamics,* 1972, 199: 311–317.

8. Hohnadel, D., et al. "Atomic absorption spectrometry of nickel, copper, zinc, lead in sweat collected from healthy subjects during sauna bathing." *Clinical Chemistry,* 1973, 19(11): 1288–1292.

9. Schnare, D., et al. "Evaluation of a detoxification regimen for fat stored xenobiotics." *Medical Hypotheses,* 1982, 9: 265–282.

10. Shields, M. & Ben, M. "Body burden reductions of PCBs, PBBs and chlorinated pesticides in human subjects." *AMBIO: A Journal of the Human Environment,* 1984, 13(5–6): 265–282.

11. Root, D. & Lionelli, G. "Excretion of lipophilic toxicant through the sebaceous glands: a case report." *Journal of Cutaneous & Ocular Toxicology,* 1987, 6(1): 13–17.

12. Schnare, D. & Robinson, P. "Reduction of hexachlorobenzene and polychlorinated biphenyl human body burdens." *Hexachlorobenzene: Proceedings of an International Symposium.* Lyon, France: International Agency for Research on Cancer, 1986.

13. Wisner, R.M., et al. "Neurotoxicity of toxic body burdens: relationship and treatment potentials." *Proceedings of International Conference on Peripheral Nerve Toxicity.* Kanasawa, Japan, 1993: 49–50.

14. Tretjak, Z., et al. "PCB reduction and clinical improvement by detoxification: an unexploited approach?" *Human & Experimental Toxicology,* 1990, 9: 235–244.

15. Kilburn, K. & Shields, M. "Neurobehavioral dysfunction in firemen exposed to polychlorinated biphenyls: possible improvement after detoxification." *Archives of Environmental Health,* 1989, 44(6): 345–349.

16. Beckmann, S., et al. "Treatment of pesticide-exposed patients with the Hubbard

method of detoxification." American Public Health Association National Conference, Washington, D.C., 1992.

17. Beckmann, S. & Tennant, F. "Precipitation of cocaine metabolites in sweat and urine of addicts undergoing sauna bath treatment." Research Center for Dependency Disorders and Chronic Pain, West Covina, Cal., 1995.

18. Wisner, R.M. & Shields, M. "Treatment of children with the detoxification method developed by Hubbard." American Academy of Environmental Medicine National Conference, Los Angeles, Cal., 1995.

19. Wisner, R.M., et al. "Human contamination and detoxification: medical response to an expanding global problem." United Nations Man and His Biosphere Programme, Moscow, 1989.

20. Root, D., et al. "Diagnosis and treatment of patients presenting subclinical signs and symptoms of exposure to chemicals which bioaccumulate in human tissue." Proceedings of the National Conference on Hazardous Wastes and Environmental Emergencies, Cincinnati, Ohio, 1985, p. 151.

21. Look Who's Coming

1. Jansson, E. "Rates skyrocket in 15 years." *Birth Defect Prevention News,* Fall 1988. Washington, D.C.: National Network to Prevent Birth Defects.

2. Jansson, E. *Components of a National Program to Reduce Birth Defect, Learning Disability, Very Low Birth Weight, and Child Abuse Rates by 50 percent and Childhood Cancer by 30 Percent.* Washington, D.C.: National Network to Prevent Birth Defects, October 21, 1987.

3. Reuben, C. *The Healthy Baby Book.* New York: Jeremy P. Tarcher, Perigee, 1992, pp. 23–26.

4. Barnes, B., et al. "Nutrition and pre-conception care (letter)." *The Lancet,* December 7, 1985, 1297.

5. Chez, R.A. "Symposium: why it's important to help patients prepare for pregnancy." *Contemporary OB/GYN,* June 1989, 33(6): 2.

6. Moos, M.K. & Cefalo, R.C. "Preconceptional health promotion: a focus for obstetric care." *American Journal of Perinatology,* January 1987, 4(1): 63.

7. See note 3 above.

8. Ibid., pp. 58–64.

9. Weathersbee, P.S., et al. "Caffeine and pregnancy: a retrospective survey." *Postgraduate Medicine,* September 1977, 62(3): 64–69.

10. Srisuphan, W. & Bracken, W. "Caffeine consumption during pregnancy and association with late spontaneous abortion." *American Journal of Obstetrics and Gynecology,* January 1986, 154: 14.

11. Goldstein, A., et al. "Passage of caffeine into human gonadal and fetal tissue." *Biochem Pharmacol,* 1962, 11: 166–168.

12. Reuben, *The Healthy Baby Book,* pp. 77–78.

13. Bracken, M. & Holford, T. "Exposure to prescribed drugs in pregnancy and association with congenital malformations." *Obstetrics & Gynecology,* September 1981, 58(3): 336.

14. Peters, J.M. "Processed meats and risk of childhood leukemia (California, USA)." *Cancer Causes and Control,* 1994, 5: 195–202.

15. Ibid.

16. Bunin, G.R., et al. "Maternal diet and risk of astrocytic glioma in children: a report from the Childrens Cancer Group (United States and Canada). *Cancer Causes and Control,* 1994, 5: 177–187.

17. Sarasua, S. & Savitz, D.A. "Cured and broiled meat consumption in relation to childhood cancer: Denver, Colorado (United States). *Cancer Causes and Control,* 1994, 5: 141–148.

18. Ibid.

19. Preston-Martin, S., et al. "N-nitroso compounds and childhood brain tumors: a case-control study." *Cancer Research,* 1982, 42: 520–524.

20. Lowengart, R.A., et al. "Childhood leukemia and parent's occupational and home exposures." *Journal of the National Cancer Institute,* 1987, 79: 39–46.

21. Deane, M., et al. "Adverse pregnancy outcomes in relation to water consumption: a re-analysis of data from the original Santa Clara County study, California, 1980–1981." *Epidemiology,* March 1992, 3(2): 94–97.

22. Wrensch, M., et al. "Spontaneous abortions and birth defects related to tap and bottled water use, San Jose, California, 1980–1985." *Epidemiology,* March 1992, 3(2): 98–103.

23. Lybarger, J., director, Division of Health Studies, Agency for Toxic Substances and Disease Registry, Public Health Service, United States Department of Health and Human Services. Testimony before the Senate Subcommittee on Superfund, Recycling, and Solid Waste Management, April 12, 1993.

24. Elkington, J. *The Poisoned Womb.* New York: Viking Penguin, 1986, pp. 48–64.

25. Ibid.

26. Ibid.

27. Joffe, J.M. "Influence of drug exposure of the father on perinatal outcome." *Clinics in Perinatology,* March 1979, 6(1): 21–36.

28. Ibid.

29. Reuben, *The Healthy Baby Book,* pp. 39–45.

30. Ibid.

31. Ibid.

32. Buckley, J.D., et al. "Occupational exposures of parents of children with acute nonlymphocytic leukemia: a report from the Childrens' Cancer Study Group." *Cancer Research,* July 15, 1989, 49: 4030–4037.

33. See note 20 above.

34. Mulinare, J., et al. "Periconceptional use of multivitamins and the occurrence of neural tube defects." *Journal of the American Medical Association,* December 2, 1988, 260, 21: 3141.

35. Peer, L.A., et al. "Effect of vitamins on human teratology." *Plastic and Reconstructive Surgery,* October 1964, 34(4): 358.

36. Tolarova, M. "Periconceptional supplementation with vitamins and folic acid to prevent recurrence of cleft lip." *The Lancet,* July 24, 1982, 2(8291): 217.

37. Committee on Evaluation of the Safety of Fishery Products. *Seafood Safety.* [ed. Ahmed, F.E.]. Washington, D.C.: National Academy Press, 1991.

22. You Are What You Eat—And Then Some

1. Tretjak, Z. "Occupational, environmental, and public health in Semic: a case study of polychlorinated biphenyl (PCB) pollution." Environmental Programs and Projects: Proceedings/Environmental Impact Analysis Research Council, 1989: 57–72.
2. Tretjak, Z. "PCB reduction and clinical improvement by detoxification: an unexploited approach." *Human and Experimental Toxicology,* 1990, 9: 235–244.

23. Save Your Waistline While Poisons Miss the Mark

1. Weissman, J. *Choose to Live.* New York: Penguin Books, 1988.
2. Tapley, D., et al. *The Columbia University College of Physicians and Surgeons: Complete Home Medical Guide.* New York: Crown Publishers, 1985, pp. 293–294.
3. Eramus, U. *Fats and Oils.* Burnaby, B.C., Canada: Alive Books, 1986.
4. Anonymous. "Got them low-fat, polyunsaturated blues." *Science News,* September 2, 1995, 148: 153.
5. Lipscomb, G. & Duggan, R. "Dietary intake of pesticide chemicals in the U.S." *Pesticides Monitoring Journal,* 1969, 2: 162–169.
6. Cornelliussen, P. "Pesticides residues in total diet samples." *Pesticides Monitoring Journal,* 1969, 5: 313–330.
7. Regenstein, L. *How To Survive in America the Poisoned.* New York: Acropolis Books, 1982, p. 273.
8. Robbins, J. *Diet For A New America.* Walpole, N.H.: Stillpoint Publishing, 1987.
9. See note 1 above.
10. See note 5 above.
11. Harris, S. "Organochlorine contamination of breast milk." Washington, D.C.: Environmental Defense Fund, 1979.
12. Carson, R. *Silent Spring.* Boston: Houghton Mifflin Co., 1962, pp. 25–26.
13. Anonymous. "Dioxin." *The Green Guide.* New York: Mothers and Others for a Livable Planet, 1995, 1
14. Duggan, R. "Dietary intake of pesticide chemicals in the United States." *Pesticides Monitoring Journal,* 1968, 2: 140–152.

24. Eat It—*Organic*

1. Mergentine, K. & Emerich, M. "Organic sales jump over $2 billion mark in 1994." *Natural Foods Merchandiser,* June 1995.
2. Anonymous. "Organic farming goes big time." *Environmental Health Perspectives,* May 1994, 102(5): 429.
3. Smith, B. "Organic foods vs. supermarket foods: element level." *Journal of Applied Nutrition,* 1993, 45(1).
4. Ibid.
5. Abell, A., et al. "High sperm density among members of organic farmers' association." *The Lancet,* June 11, 1994, 343: 1498.

6. Knorr, D. "Quality of ecologically grown food." *Cereal Foods World,* 1982, 27(4): 165–167.

7. *IARC Monographs,* 1986, 41: 357–406.

8. Hoar, S.K., et al. "Agricultural herbicide use and risk of lymphoma and soft-tissue sarcoma." *Journal of the American Medical Association,* 1986, 256: 1141–1147.

9. Woods, J.S., et al. "Soft tissue sarcoma and non-Hodgkin's lymphoma in relation to phenoxy herbicide and chlorinated phenol exposure in western Washington." *Journal of the National Cancer Institute,* 1987, 78: 899–910.

10. Balarajan, R. & Acheson, E.D. "Soft tissue sarcomas in agriculture and forestry workers." *Journal of Epidemiology and Community Health,* 1984, 38: 113–116.

11. Anonymous. "Shoppers seeking out organic produce." *The Wall Street Journal,* September 23, 1994, B1.

12. Baker, B. & McGee, P. "CDFA pesticide residue analysis of organics. A special CCOF report." *California Certified Organic Farmers State Newsletter,* Fall 1991, 8(4): 6.

13. Steinman, D. *Diet for a Poisoned Planet.* New York: Ballantine Books, 1992, p. 326.

14. National Research Council. *Pesticides in the Diets of Infants and Children.* Washington, D.C.: National Academy Press, 1993.

15. Wiles, R. & Campbell, C. *Pesticides in Children's Food.* Washington, D.C.: Environmental Working Group, 1993.

16. Steinman, D. & Epstein, S.S. *The Safe Shopper's Bible.* New York: Macmillan, 1995, pp. 295–307.

25. Something Fishy

1. Steinman, D. *Diet for a Poisoned Planet.* New York: Ballantine Books, 1992, p. 104.

2. Leaf, A. "Cardiovascular effects of fish oils—beyond the platelet." *Circulation,* 1990, 82: 624–628.

3. Shekelle, R.B., et al. "Fish and coronary heart disease: the epidemiologic evidence." *Nutrition, Metabolism and Cardiovascular Disease,* 1993, 3: 46–51.

4. Kromhout, D., et al. "The inverse relation between fish consumption and 20 year mortality from coronary heart disease." *The New England Journal of Medicine,* 1985, 312: 1205–1209.

5. Shekelle, R.B., et al. "Fish consumption and mortality from coronary heart disease." *The New England Journal of Medicine,* 1985, 313: 820.

6. Dolecek, T.A. & Grandits, G. "Dietary polyunsaturated fatty acids and mortality in the multiple risk factor intervention trial (MRFIT)." *World Review of Nutrition and Dietetics,* 1991, 66: 205–216.

7. Kromhout, D., et al. "The protective effect of a small amount of fish on coronary heart disease mortality in an elderly population." *International Journal of Epidemiology,* 1995, 24: 340–345.

8. Epstein, S.S. & Steinman, D. "All we're doing is rearranging the deck chairs on a seafood titanic." *Los Angeles Times,* February 18, 1994.

9. Gossett, R., et al. "Human serum DDT levels related to consumption of fish from the coastal waters of Los Angeles—*short communication.*" *Environmental Toxicology and Chemistry,* 1989, 8(10): 951–955.

10. Committee on Evaluation of the Safety of Fishery Products. *Seafood Safety.* [ed. Ahmed, F.E.]. Washington, D.C.: National Academy Press, 1991.

11. Ibid.

12. Wasserman, M., et al. "Organochlorine compounds in neoplastic and adjacent apparently normal breast tissue." *Bulletin of Environmental Contamination and Toxicology,* 1976, 15: 478–484.

13. Mussalo-Rauhamaa, H.E., et al. "Occurrence of beta-hexachlorocyclohexane in breast cancer patients." *Cancer,* 1990, 66: 2124–2128.

14. Falck, F.A., et al. "Pesticides and polychlorinated biphenyl residues in human breast lipids and their relation to breast cancer." *Archives of Environmental Health,* 1992, 47: 143–146.

15. Wolff, M., et al. "Blood levels of organochlorine residues and risk of breast cancer." *Journal of the National Cancer Institute,* 1993, 85(8): 648–652.

16. Wolff, M.S. & Toniolo, P.G. "Correspondence." *Journal of the National Cancer Institute,* 1994, 86(14): 1095–1096.

17. Salonen, J.T., et al. "Intake of mercury from fish, lipid peroxidation, and the risk of myocardial infarction and coronary, cardiovascular, and any death in eastern Finnish men." *Circulation,* 1995; 91(3): 645–655.

18. Ngim, C.H. & Devathasan, G. "Epidemiologic study on the association between body burden mercury level and idiopathic Parkinson's disease." *Neuroepidemiology,* 1989, 8: 128–141.

19. Fein, G.G., et al. "Prenatal exposure to polychlorinated biphenyls: effects of birth size and gestational age." *Journal of Pediatrics,* 1984, 106: 315–320.

20. Jacobson, S.W., et al. "The effect of intrauterine PCB exposure on visual recognition memory." *Child Development,* 1985, 56: 853–860.

21. Jacobson, J.L., et al. "Effects of *in utero* exposure to polychlorinated biphenyls and related contaminants on cognitive functioning in young children." *Journal of Pediatrics,* 1990, 116: 38–45.

22. Daly, H.B. "The evaluation of behavioral changes produced by consumption of environmentally contaminated fish." *The Vulnerable Brain and Environmental Risks. Volume 1. Malnutrition and Hazard Assessment.* [eds. Isaacson, R.L. & Jensen, K.F.]. New York: Plenum Press, 1992, pp. 151–171.

23. Anonymous. "Got them low-fat, polyunsaturated blues." *Science News,* September 2, 1995, 148: 153.

24. See note 9 above.

26. How Sweet It Isn't

1. Blaylock, R. *Excitotoxins.* Santa Fe: Health Press, 1995, p. 211.

2. Lawlor, P. *Sweet Talk: Media Coverage of Artificial Sweeteners.* Washington, D.C.: The Media Institute, 1986.

3. "America's sweet tooth." Washington, D.C.: United States Department of Agriculture, 1984, 50, 184.

4. McCann, M., et al. "Non-calorie sweeteners and weight reduction." *Journal of American Dietary Association,* 1956, 32: 337–330.

5. Rosenman, K. "Benefits of saccharin: a review." *Environmental Research,* 1978, 15: 70–81.

6. Adams, G., et al. "Weight loss: long term results in an ambulatory setting." *Journal of American Dietary Association,* 1983, 83: 306–310.

7. Finer, N. "Sugar substitutes in the treatment of obesity and diabetes mellitus." *Clinical Nutrition,* 1985, 4: 207–214.

8. Roberts, H. "A clinician's adventures in medicine: is aspartame (Nutrasweet) safe?" *On Call.* Palm Beach, Fla.: Palm Beach County Medical Society, 1987, p. 16.

9. Wurtman, R. "Aspartame: possible effects on seizure susceptibility." *The Lancet,* 1986, 1060.

10. Walton, R. "Seizure and mania after high intake of aspartame." *Psychosomatics,* 1986, 27: 218–220.

11. Roberts, H. "Dry eyes from use of aspartame (Nutrasweet): associated insights concerning the sjogren syndrome." *Townsend Letter for Doctors,* 1994: 82–83.

12. Gonda, A., et al. "Hemodialysis for methanol intoxication." *American Journal of Medicine,* 1978, 64: 749–757.

13. McMartin, K., et al. "Methanol poisoning in humans: role of formic acid accumulation in metabolic acidosis." *American Journal of Medicine,* 1980, 68: 414–418.

14. Remington, D. "FDA approval of aspartame." Twenty-third Annual Meeting, American Academy of Environmental Medicine, Lake Tahoe, Nevada, 1989.

15. "Facts you should know about aspartame or Nutrasweet." Ocala, Fla.: Aspartame Victims & Their Friends.

27. Water, Water Everywhere and Not a Drop to Drink

1. Houk, V.N. cited in *Pesticides and Groundwater: A Health Concern for the Midwest.* Navarre, Minn.: Freshwater Foundation, March 1988, pp. 221–222.

2. *The Clean Water Act 20 Years Later.* New York: Island Press and the Natural Resources Defense Council.

3. Ibid.

4. Olson, E. *Think Before You Drink.* New York: Natural Resources Defense Council, September 1993, p. 3.

5. Ibid., p. i.

6. Ibid., p. 4.

7. Morris, R.D., et al. "Chlorination, chlorination by-products, and cancer: a meta-analysis." *American Journal of Public Health,* 1992, 82(7): 955–963.

8. Olson, *Think Before You Drink,* p. iv.

9. Ibid., p. v.

10. Brown, J.P., et al. University of California at Berkeley and California Environmental Protection Agency, review of arsenic in drinking water studies, referenced in *Science News,* April 1992, p. 253.

11. United States Environmental Protection Agency. *Addendum To: The Occurrence and Exposure Assessments for Radon, Radium 226, Radium 228, Uranium, and Gross Alpha Particle Activity in Public Drinking Water Supplies.* September 30, 1992.

12. "Proposed radionuclide rules." 56 *Federal Register* at 33067, 33076, 33082 (1991): Comments of the National Resources Defense Council, et al., on EPA's Proposed NPDWRs for radionuclide (November 1991).

13. Jackson, R.J. "DBCP and drinking water in California." *Pesticides and Groundwater:*

A Health Concern in the Midwest. Proceedings of a conference held October 16–17, 1986. Navarre, Minn.: Freshwater Foundation.

14. King, J. *Troubled Water.* Emmaus, Pa.: Rodale Press, 1985, p. 57.

15. Manning, A. "Tainted water. Herbicide levels rise in summer." *USA Today,* August 18, 1995, D1.

16. Fagliano, J., et al. "Drinking water contamination and the incidence of leukemia: an ecologic study." *American Journal of Public Health,* 1990, 80(10): 1209–1212.

17. Needleman, H.L., et al. "Deficits in psychological and classroom performance of children with congenital anomalies." *Journal of the American Medical Association,* June 8, 1984, 251: 689–695.

18. Deane, M., et al. "Adverse pregnancy outcomes in relation to water consumption: a re-analysis of data from the original Santa Clara County study, California, 1980–1981." *Epidemiology,* March 1992, 3(2): 94–97.

19. Wrensch, M., et al. "Spontaneous abortions and birth defects related to tap and bottled water use, San Jose, California, 1980–1985." *Epidemiology,* March 1992, 3(2): 98–103.

20. Ibid.

21. See note 15 above.

22. Wiles, R., et al. *Tap Water Blues: Herbicides in Drinking Water.* Washington, D.C.: Environmental Working Group, 1994, p. 106.

23. Anonymous. "Is lead a problem in my drinking water?" Washington, D.C.: League of Women Voters Education Fund, undated.

24. Anonymous. "Study finds contaminants in bottled water." *Water Technology,* June 1987, 35.

25. Lefferts, L.F. & Schmidt, S.B. "Water: safe to swallow?" *Nutrition Action Health Letter,* November 1988, 15(9): 1, 5–7.

26. *Epid. Infec.,* 1987, 99: 439.

27. Hernandez, D.H. and Rosenberg, F.A. "Antibiotic-resistant pseudomonas in bottled drinking water." *Canadian Journal of Microbiology,* April 1987, 33: 286–289.

28. You Make Me So Excited . . .

1. Blaylock, R. *Excitotoxins: The Taste That Kills.* Santa Fe, N.M.: Health Press, 1995.

2. Olney, J. "Excitotoxic food additives: functional teratological aspects." In *Progress in Brain Research.* New York: Elevier Science Publications, 1988.

3. Reinis, S. & Goldman, J. "The development of the brain." *Biological and Functional Perspectives.* Springfield, Ill.: Thomas Books, 1980, pp. 211–213.

4. Olney, J. "Glutamate, a neurotoxic transmitter." *Journal of Child Neurology,* 1989, 4: 218–225.

5. Lucas, D. & Newhouse, J. "The toxic effect of sodium L-glutamate on the inner layers of the retina." *Archives of Ophthalmology,* 1957, 58: 193–201.

6. Olney, J. "Brain lesions, obesity, and other disturbances in mice treated with monosodium glutamate." *Science,* 1969, 165: 719–721.

7. Olney, J. "Toxic effects of glutamate and related amino acids on the developing central nervous system." *Heritable Disorders of Amino Acid Metabolism.* [Nylan, W.N., ed.]. New York: John Wiley, 1974.

8. Olney, J. "Glutamate, a neurotoxic transmitter." *Journal of Child Neurology,* 1989, 4: 218–226.
9. See note 4 above.
10. See note 1 above.
11. Mattson, M. "Antigenic changes to those seen in neurofibrillary tangles are elicited by glutamate and Ca + 2 influx in cultured hippocampal neurons." *Neurology,* 1990, 2: 105–117.
12. Olney, J. & deGubareff. "Glutamate neurotoxicity and Huntington's chorea." *Nature,* 1978, 271: 557–559.
13. Olney, J. & Zorumski, C. "Excitotoxicity of L-dopa and 6-OH-DOPA: implications for Parkinson's and Huntington's diseases." *Experimental Neurology,* 1990, 108: 269–272.

29. Grow Your Own

1. The Earth Works Group. *The Next Step: 50 More Things You Can Do to Save the Earth.* Kansas City, Mo.: Andrews & McMeel, Universal Press Syndicate Group, 1991, p. 72.
2. Mowrey, D. *The Scientific Validation of Herbal Medicine.* New Canaan, Conn.: Keats Publishing, 1986, pp. 91–92.
3. Hoffman, D. *The New Holistic Herbal.* Rockport, Mass.: Element, 1990, p. 196.
4. Ibid., p. 222.
5. Ibid., p. 202.
6. Ibid., p. 210.
7. Mowrey, *The Scientific Validation of Herbal Medicine,* p. 243.
8. Ibid., p. 279.
9. Ibid., pp. 178–179.
10. See note 3 above.
11. Ibid.
12. Mattern, V. "Food you can grow in the shade." *Organic Gardening,* April 1995, 70–76.

30. Feminizing Jake

1. Bulger, W.H. & Kupfer, D. "Estrogenic activity of pesticides and other xenobiotics on the uterus and male reproductive tract." *Endocrine Toxicology.* [eds: Thomas, J.A., et al.]. New York: Raven Press, 1985, pp. 1–33.
2. Colborn, T., et al. "Development effects of endocrine-disrupting chemicals in wild-life and humans." *Environmental Health Perspectives,* October 1993, 101(5): 378–384.
3. Auger, J., et al. "Decline in semen quality among fertile men in Paris during the past 20 years." *The New England Journal of Medicine,* February 2, 1995, 332(5): 281–285.
4. See note 2 above.
5. Sharpe, R.M. & Skakkebaek, N.E. "Are oestrogens involved in falling sperm counts and disorders of the male reproductive tract?" *The Lancet,* May 29, 1993, 341: 1392–1395.

6. Giwercman, A. & Skakkebaek, N.E. "The human testis—an organ at risk?" *International Journal of Andrology,* 1992, 15: 373–375.

7. Jackson, M.B. "John Radcliffe Hospital Cryptorchidism Research Group. The epidemiology of cryptorchidism." *Hormone Research,* 1988, 30: 153–156.

8. Osterlind, A. "Diverging trends in incidence and mortality of testicular cancer in Denmark, 1943–1982." *British Journal of Cancer,* 1986, 53: 501–505.

9. Waller, D.P., et al. "Physiology and toxicology of the male reproductive tract." *Endocrine Toxicology.* [ed. Thomas, J.A., et al.]. New York: Raven Press, 1985, pp. 269–333.

10. Chilvers, C., et al. "Apparent doubling of frequency of undescended testis in England and Wales in 1962–81." *The Lancet,* 1984, ii: 330–332.

11. Anonymous. "Testicular descent revisited." (Editorial.) *The Lancet,* 1989; i: 360–361.

12. See note 6 above.

13. Soto, A.M., et al. "P-nonyl-phenol: an estrogenic xenobiotic released from 'modified' polystyrene." *Environmental Health Perspectives,* 1991, 92: 167–173.

14. Krishnan, A.V., et al. "Bisphenol-A: an estrogenic substance is released from polycarbonate flasks during autoclaving." *Endocrinology,* 1993, 132: 2279–2286.

31. You've Come a Long Way, Baby . . . or Have You?

1. Gibbons, A. "Dioxin tied to endometriosis." *Science,* November 26, 1993, 262: 1373.

2. Ibid.

3. Ibid.

4. Donna, A., et al. "Ovarian mesothelial tumors and herbicides: a case-control study." *Carcinogenesis,* 1984; 5(7): 941–942.

5. Donna, A., et al. "Triazine herbicides and ovarian epithelian neoplasms." *Scandinavian Journal of Work, Environment and Health,* 1989; 15: 47–53.

6. Wasserman, M., et al. "Organochlorine compounds in neoplastic and adjacent apparently normal breast tissue." *Bulletin of Environmental Contamination and Toxicology,* 1976, 15: 478–484.

7. Mussalo-Rauhamaa, H.E., et al. "Occurrence of beta-hexachlorocyclhexane in breast cancer patients." *Cancer,* 1990, 66: 2124–2128.

8. Falck, F.A., et al. "Pesticides and polychlorinated biphenyl residues in human breast lipids and their relation to breast cancer." *Archives of Environmental Health,* 1992, 47: 143–146.

9. Wolff, M., et al. "Blood levels of organochlorine residues and risk of breast cancer." *Journal of the National Cancer Institute,* 1993, 85(8): 648–652.

10. Wolff, M.S. & Toniolo, P.G. "Correspondence." *Journal of the National Cancer Institute,* 1994, 86(14): 1095–1096.

11. Gaskill, S.P., et al. "Breast cancer mortality and diet in the United States." *Cancer Research,* 1979, 39: 3628–3637.

12. Armstrong, B. & Doll, R. "Environmental factors and cancer incidence and mortality in different countries, with special reference to dietary practices." *International Journal of Cancer,* 1975, 15: 617–631.

13. Segi, M., et al. "The relation between food patterns and the death rates for stomach cancer and the cancer of the intestine and breast by countries." Nagoya, Japan: Segi Institute of Cancer Epidemiology, 1977.

14. Stocks, P. "Breast cancer anomalies." *British Journal of Cancer,* 1970, 24: 633–643.

15. Hirayama, T. "Epidemiology of breast cancer with special reference to the role of diet." *Preventive Medicine,* 1978, 7: 173–195.

16. Phillips, R.L. "Role of life-style and dietary habits in risk of cancer among Seventh-Day Adventists." *Cancer Research,* 1975, 35: 3513–3522.

17. Adlercreutz, H., et al., "Urinary excretion of lignans and isoflavonoid phytoestrogens in Japanese men and women consuming a traditional Japanese diet." *American Journal of Clinical Nutrition,* 1991, 54: 1093–1100.

18. Adlercreutz, H, et al. "Dietary phyto-oestrogens and the menopause in Japan." *The Lancet,* May 16, 1992, 339: 1233.

19. Cassidy, A., et al. "Biological effects of a diet of soy protein rich in isoflavones on the menstrual cycle of premenopausal women." *American Journal of Clinical Nutrition,* 1994, 60: 333–340.

20. Liu, H., et al. "Indolo[3,2-b]carbazole: a dietary-derived factor that exhibits both antiestrogenic and estrogenic activity." *Journal of the National Cancer Institute,* December 7, 1994, 86(23): 1758–1765.

21. Lefferts, L.Y. "Limiting hormone-altering chemicals." *The Green Guide,* 1995, 15: 1–3.

33. I Have One Word for You—Plastic

1. "Styrene: health effects of low-level exposure." *FASE Reports,* 1988, 7(2): 1, 10.

2. Boillat, M., et al. *Soz. Prevent.* 1986, 31: 260–262.

3. Rosen, I., et al. *Scandinavian Journal of Work, Environment and Health,* 1978, 4: 184–194.

4. Cherry, N., et al. *British Journal of Industrial Medicine,* 1981, 38: 346–350.

5. Gamberale, F., et al. *Scandinavian Journal of Work, Environment and Health,* 1972, 11: 86–93.

6. Gorell, P., et al. *Scandinavian Journal of Work, Environment and Health,* 1972, 9: 76–83.

7. Mackay, C., et al. *Human Toxicology,* 1986, 5: 85–89.

8. Mutti, A., et al. *American Journal of Industrial Medicine,* 1984, 5: 275–284.

9. Harkonen, H. *International Archives of Occupational and Environmental Health,* 1977, 46: 231–239.

10. Lilis, R., et al. *Environmental Research,* 1978, 15: 133–138.

11. Sappalainen, A., et al. *Scandinavian Journal of Work, Environment and Health,* 1976, 3: 140–146.

12. Rousseau, D., et al. *Your Home Your Health & Your Well-Being.* Berkeley, Cal.: Ten Speed Press, 1988, p. 73.

13. Raloff, J. "Plastics may shed chemical estrogens." *Science News,* 1993, 144: 12.

34. Wax Your Car, Not Your Tummy

1. *The Wax Coverup: What Consumers Aren't Told About Pesticides on Fresh Produce.* Washington, D.C.: Americans for Safe Food; Center for Science in the Public Interest, Washington D.C.

2. Anonymous. "FDA spells out labeling for pesticide-treated, coated produce." *Food Chemical News,* 1989, 8–9.

3. 21 CFR 101.100 (a) (2) Section 403 (I) (2) Federal Food, Drug, and Cosmetic Act (FFDCA).

4. "Petition Proposing Revocation of Food Additive Tolerances." *Federal Register,* 1989, 54(125): 27701.

5. Klaasen, C., et al. *Casarett and Doull's Toxicology.* New York: Macmillan, 1986, p. 563.

6. Mott, L. & Snyder, K. *Pesticide Alert: A Guide to Pesticides in Fruits and Vegetables.* San Francisco: Sierra Club Books, 1987, p. 64.

7. Klaasen, C., et al., *Casarett and Doull's Toxicology,* p. 258.

8. International Agency for Research on Cancer. *IARC Monographs on the Evaluation of Carcinogenic Risks to Humans,* Supplement 7. Lyon, France: World Health Organization, 1987, 71, 392.

35. Snow White Has a Black Heart

1. Raloff, J. "Dioxin: paper's trace, chlorine bleaching of wood pulp appears to leave a toxic legacy in much of the paper we encounter." *Science News.*

2. Ibid.

3. Bertazzi, P., et al. *Epidemiology,* 1993, 4: 398.

4. Fingerhut, M., et al. *New England Journal of Medicine,* 1991, 324: 212.

5. Kogevinas, M., et al. *Cancer Causes and Control,* 1993, 4: 547.

6. Manz, A., et al. *The Lancet,* 1991, 338: 959.

7. Zober, A., et al. *International Archives of Occupational and Environmental Health,* 1990, 62: 139.

8. Environmental Protection Agency. *Broad Scan Analysis of the FY82 National Human Adipose Tissue Survey Specimens,* Vol. I, Washington, D.C.: Office of Toxic Substances, 1986, EPA-560/5-86-035.

9. Orban, J., et al. "Dioxin and dibenzofurans in adipose tissue of general U.S. population and selected subpopulations." *American Journal of Public Health,* 1994, 84: 439–450.

10. "Pointing the finger at chlorine." Washington, D.C.: *Greenpeace,* 1995, 4(1): 1.

11. *The Village Voice,* New York: 1995.

12. Lee, G. "Getting some answers on potential killer: EPA report to detail risks from dioxin." *Washington Post,* June 14, 1994.

13. Gibbons, A. "Dioxin tied to endometriosis." *Science,* 1994, 1373.

14. See note 3 above.

15. See note 4 above.

16. See note 6 above.

17. Regenstein, L. *How To Survive in America the Poisoned.* New York: Acropolis Books, 1982, p. 298.

18. *Chemosphere,* January 1988.

19. Norland, R. & Friedman, J. "Poison at our doorstep." *Philadelphia Inquirer,* September 23–28, 1979.

20. *Environmental Science and Technology,* 1991.

21. "Four priorities: ending chlorine poisoning." Washington, D.C.: *Greenpeace,* 1995, 4(1): 4.

36. There Goes the Ozone

1. Al Gore cited in *Ozone.* Washington, D.C.: *Greenpeace* (undated).
2. Leaf, A. "Ozone depletion and public health." *Hospital Practice,* June 15, 1994, 9–10.
3. Lieberman, J. "Adequacy of protection sunglasses and sunscreens." Testimony before Ad Hoc Subcommittee on Consumer and Environmental Issues of the Committee on Governmental Affairs, United States Senate, One Hundred Second Congress, Second, June 5, 1992. Washington, D.C.: Government Printing Office, 1993, p. 1.
4. Kripke, M.L. "Adequacy of protection sunglasses and sunscreens." Testimony before Ad Hoc Subcommittee on Consumer and Environmental Issues of the Committee on Governmental Affairs, United States Senate, One Hundred Second Congress, Second, June 5, 1992. Washington, D.C.: Government Printing Office, 1993, p. 9.
5. Ibid., p. 8.
6. Grant-Kels, J.M. "Adequacy of protection sunglasses and sunscreens." Testimony before Ad Hoc Subcommittee on Consumer and Environmental Issues of the Committee on Governmental Affairs, United States Senate, One Hundred Second Congress, Second, June 5, 1992. Washington, D.C.: Government Printing Office, 1993, pp. 10–11.
7. De Fabo, E.G. "Adequacy of protection sunglasses and sunscreens." Testimony before Ad Hoc Subcommittee on Consumer and Environmental Issues of the Committee on Governmental Affairs, United States Senate, One Hundred Second Congress, Second, June 5, 1992. Washington, D.C.: Government Printing Office, 1993, p. 16.
8. Burke, K.E. "Oral and topical l-selenomethionine protection from ultraviolet-induced sunburn, tanning and skin cancer." *Journal of Orthomolecular Medicine,* 1992, 7(2): 83–94.
9. Murray, M. & Pizzorno, J. *Encyclopedia of Natural Medicine.* Rocklin, Cal.: Prima Publishing, 1991, pp. 192–196.

37. Voting at the Checkout Line

1. Material Safety Data Sheet. "Ajax." Colgate-Palmolive, New York, 1994.
2. *International Agency for Research on Cancer Monographs,* 1987, supplement 7, pp. 341–342.
3. Steinman, D. & Epstein, S.S. *The Safe Shopper's Bible.* New York: Macmillan, 1995, p. 69.
4. Engler, R. "List of chemicals evaluated for carcinogenic potential. " Memorandum. United States Environmental Protection Agency, Health Effects Division, October 14, 1992, p. 2.
5. Steinman, D. & Epstein, S.S. *The Safe Shopper's Bible.* New York: Macmillan, 1995 p. 34.

6. Mergentime, K. & Emerich, M. "Organic sales jump over $2 billion mark in 1994." *Natural Foods Merchandiser,* June 1995, 74–76.

38. Put a Pretty Face On

1. "Potential health hazards of cosmetic products." Hearings before the Subcommittee on Regulation and Business Opportunities of the Committee on Small Business. House of Representatives. July 14 and September 15, 1988. Washington, D.C.: United States Government Printing Office, 1989.

2. "Nitrosamine-contaminated cosmetics; call for industry action; request for data." *Federal Register,* April 10, 1979, 44(70): 21365.

3. Ibid.

4. Food and Drug Administration, Division of Colors and Cosmetics. "Progress report on the analysis of cosmetic products and raw materials for nitrosamines." March 1, 1988.

5. International Agency for Research on Cancer (IARC). *Occupational Exposures of Hairdressers and Barbers and Personal Use of Hair Colourants; Some Hair Dyes; Cosmetic Colourants, and Industrial Dyestuffs and Aromatic Amines.* Lyon, France: World Health Organization, 1993, 57: 62.

6. Bogovski, P. & Bogovski, S. "Animal species in which N-nitroso compounds induce cancer." *International Journal of Cancer,* 1981, 27: 471–474.

7. Druckrey, H., et al. "Organotrope carcinogene Wirkungen bei 65 verschiedenen N-nitroso-verbindungen an BD-ratten." *Z. Krebsorsch,* 1967, 69: 103–201.

8. Magee, P.N., et al. "N-nitroso compounds and related carcinogens." *American Chemical Society Monograph,* 1976, 173: 491–625.

9. See note 4 above.

10. Hoffmann, D. & Hecht, S.S. "Nicotine-derived N-nitrosamines and tobacco-related cancer: current status and future directions." *Cancer Research,* March 1985, 45: 935–944.

11. Ibid.

12. Ibid.

13. Preston-Martin, S., et al. "N-nitroso compounds and childhood brain tumors: a case-control study." *Cancer Research,* December 1982, 42: 5240–5245.

14. See note 5 above.

15. Thrasher, J. & Broughton, A. *The Poisoning of Our Homes & Workplaces.* Santa Ana, Cal.: Seadora, Inc., 1989.

16. Conry, T. *Consumer's Guide to Cosmetics.* Garden City, N.Y.: Anchor Press/Doubleday, 1980, p. 73.

17. Winter, R. *A Consumer's Dictionary of Cosmetic Ingredients.* New York: Crown Publishers, 1989, p. 120.

18. Kantor, G.R., et al. "Acute allergic contact dermatitis from diazolidinyl urea (Germall II) in a hair gel." *Journal of the American Academy of Dermatology,* 1985, 13: 116–119.

19. Stephens, T.J., et al. "Experimental delayed contact sensitization to diazolidinyl urea (Germall II) in guinea pigs." *Contact Dermatitis,* 1987, 16: 164–168.

20. Johansen, M. & Bundgaard, H. "Kinetics of formaldehyde release from the cosmetic preservative Germall 115. *Arch. Pharm. Chem. Sci.,* 1981, 9: 117–122.
21. Winter, R. *A Consumer's Dictionary of Cosmetic Ingredients,* p. 256.
22. Adams, R.M. & Mailbach, H.I. "A five-year study of cosmetic reactions." *Journal of the American Academy of Dermatology,* 1985, 13(6): 1062–1069.
23. Winter, R. *A Consumer's Dictionary of Cosmetic Ingredients,* p. 201.
24. Hannuksela, M. "Rapid increase in contact allergy to Kathon® CG in Finland." *Contact Dermatitis,* 1986, 15: 211–214.
25. Winter, R. *A Consumer's Dictionary of Cosmetic Ingredients,* p. 222.
26. *Natural Body Care Reports,* June 1991, 2(1): 3. Published by Earth Science, Inc., of Corona, Cal. This report discusses each of the ingredients listed.
27. Hampton, A. *Natural Organic Hair and Skin Care.* Tampa, Fla.: Organic Press, 1987.
28. Winter, R. *A Consumer's Dictionary of Cosmetic Ingredients,* p. 232.
29. See note 26 above.
30. Ibid.
31. Winter, R. *A Consumer's Dictionary of Cosmetic Ingredients,* p. 307.
32. Ibid., p. 318.
33. Ibid., p. 43.

39. I Smell a Rat

1. Wilkenfeld, I. "Perfume or pollutant?" *Green Alternatives,* November/December 1992, 32–34.
2. Winter, R. *A Consumer's Dictionary of Cosmetic Ingredients,* New York: Crown Publishers, 1989, p. 10.
3. See note 1 above.
4. *Neurotoxins: At Home and the Workplace.* Report by Committee on Science and Technology, Washington, D.C.: United States House of Representatives, 1986, 99–827.
5. Report (99–827) to United States House of Representatives, Subcommittee on Business Opportunities, National Institute of Occupational Safety and Health, Washington, D.C., September 16, 1988.
6. Kirland, D., et al. "Hair dye genotoxicity." *American Heart Association Journal,* 1979, 98: 6.
7. Wallace, L. "Twenty most common chemicals found in thirty-one fragrance products." Environmental Protection Agency, Health Hazard Information, 1991.
8. Stevens, K. "How safe are perfumes?" *The Human Ecologist,* 1990, 15.
9. Ibid.
10. Adams, R.M. & Maibach, H.I. "A five-year study of cosmetic reactions." *Journal of the American Academy of Dermatology,* 1985, 13(6): 1062–1069.
11. See note 7 above.
12. See note 8 above.
13. See note 1 above.
14. Ibid.

15. Toth, D. "Manufacturers smell success in mood-altering perfumes." *The New York Times,* 1990, C1–C2.

40. Don't Get Dirty in the Shower

1. Lybarger, J., director, Division of Health Studies, Agency for Toxic Substances and Disease Registry, Public Health Service, United States Department of Health and Human Services. Testimony before the Senate Subcommittee on Superfund, Recycling, and Solid Waste Management, April 12, 1993.
2. Environmental Protection Agency, Office of Water Planning and Standards. "Identification and evaluation of waterborne routes of exposure from other than food and drinking water." Contract No. 68-01-3857, January 1979.
3. Brown, H., et al. "The role of skin absorption as a route of exposure for volatile organic compounds in drinking water." *American Journal of Public Health,* 1984, 74: 479–484.
4. Andelman, J.B. "Human exposures to volatile halogenated organic chemicals in indoor and outdoor air." *Environmental Health Perspective,* 1985, 62: 313–318.
5. Ibid.

41. A Smile That Won't Kill You

1. "Is there poison in your mouth?" *60 Minutes.* New York: CBS News, December 16, 1990.
2. Treptow, R.S. "Amalgam dental fillings, parts I and II." *Chemistry,* April 17–20, May 15–19, 1978.
3. See note 1 above.
4. Ibid.
5. Huggins, H.A. *PAR: Proper Amalgam Removal.* Colorado Springs: Huggins Diagnostic Center, 1993, p. 9.
6. See note 1 above.
7. Pleva, J. "Corrosion and mercury release from dental amalgam." *Journal of Orthomolecular Medicine,* 1989, 4(3): 141–158.
8. See note 1 above.
9. Halbach, S. "Amalgam tooth fillings and man's mercury burden." *Human and Experimental Toxicology,* 1994, 13: 496–501.
10. Huggins, H.A. "Mercury: a factor in mental disease?" *The Journal of Orthomolecular Psychiatry,* 1982, 11(1): 3–16.
11. Ngim, C.H & Devathasan, G. "Epidemiologic study on the association between body burden mercury level and idiopathic Parkinson's disease." *Neuroepidemiology,* 1989, 8: 128–141.
12. Wenstrup, D., et al. "Trace element imbalances in isolated subcellular fractions of Alzheimer's disease brains." *Brain research,* 1990, 553: 125–131.
13. See note 10 above.
14. Zamm, A.V. "Removal of dental mercury: often an effective treatment for the very sensitive patient." *Journal of Orthomolecular Medicine,* 1990, 5(3): 138–142.

15. Kristal, H.J. "Protocol for mercury and nickel toxicity." *Townsend Letter for Doctors*, February/March 1992, 154.
16. Huggins, H.A. *PAR: Proper Amalgam Removal*, p. 32.

42. Hair Dyes to Die For

1. Anonymous. "Are hair dyes safe?" *Consumer Reports*, August 1979, 456–460.
2. International Agency for Research on Cancer. *IARC Monographs on the Evaluation of Carcinogenic Risks to Humans. Occupational Exposures of Hairdressers and Barbers and Personal Use of Hair Colourants; Some Hair Dyes, Cosmetic Colourants, Industrial Dyestuffs and Aromatic Amines.* Volume 57. Lyon, France, 1993.
3. See note 1 above.
4. Markowitz, J.A., et al. "Hair dyes and acute nonlymphocytic leukemia (ANLL)." *American Journal of Epidemiology*, 1985, 122: 523. Abstract.
5. Cantor, K.P., et al. "Hair dye use and risk of leukemia and lymphoma." *American Journal of Public Health*, 1988, 78: 570–571.
6. Zahm, S., et al. "Use of hair coloring products and the risk of lymphoma, multiple myeloma, and chronic lymphocytic leukemia." *American Journal of Public Health*, 1992, 82(7): 990–997.
7. Brown, L.M., et al. "Hair dye use and multiple myeloma in white men." *American Journal of Public Health*, 1992, 82: 1673–1674.
8. See note 2 above.
9. Thun, M.J., et al. "Hair dye use and risk of fatal cancers in U.S. women." *Journal of the National Cancer Institute*, 1994, 86(3): 210–215.
10. See note 7 above.
11. See note 4 above.
12. See note 5 above.
13. See note 6 above.
14. International Agency for Research on Cancer. *IARC Monographs on the Evaluation of the Carcinogenic Risks to Humans. Overall Evaluations of Carcinogenicity: An Updating of IARC Monographs Volumes 1 to 42.* Lyon, France: World Health Organization, 1987, pp. 230–232.
15. Steinman, D. & Epstein, S.S. *The Safe Shopper's Bible.* New York: Macmillan, 1995, pp. 182, 240–244, 417–418.
16. Kuijten, R.R., et al. "Parental occupation and childhood astrocytoma: results of a case-control study." *Cancer Research*, 1992, 52: 782–786.
17. Kramer, S., et al. "Medical and drug risk factors associated with neuroblastoma: a case-control study." *Journal of the National Cancer Institute*, 1987, 78: 797–804.
18. Bunin, G.R., et al. "Gestational risk factors for Wilms' tumor: results of a case-control study." *Cancer Research*, 1987, 47: 2972–2977.
19. See note 15 above.
20. Nisbet, I.C.T. & Rosenblatt, K. "Carcinogenic risk estimates for 2,4-DAA." A report prepared by Clement Associates, Inc., nondated, p. 22.
21. Ibid.

43. The All-American Road Race . . . Hold Your Breath!

1. Surman, B. "Worst pollutants found indoors, scientists say." *Los Angeles Times,* September 11, 1986, 26.
2. "In-vehicle air toxics." Los Angeles, California: South Coast Air Quality Management District: 3.
3. Ibid.
4. Elkington, J., Hailes, J. & Makower, J. *The Green Consumer.* New York: Penguin Books, 1990, p. 22.
5. Pepelko, W. & Peirano, W. "Health effects of exposure to diesel engine emissions." *Journal of the American College of Toxicology,* 1983, 2(4): 253–306.
6. See note 1 above.
7. Sittig, M. *Handbook of Toxic and Hazardous Chemicals and Carcinogens.* Park Ridge, N.J.: Noyes Publications, 1985, pp. 111–113, 422–426, 868–869, 931–932.

44. You Can't Get That Raise . . . If You're Not Alive

1. Sittig, M. *Handbook of Toxic and Hazardous Chemicals and Carcinogens.* Park Ridge, N.J.: Noyes Publications, 1985, pp. 462–464.
2. Sterling, T. & Arundel, A. "Formaldehyde and lung cancer." *The Lancet,* 1985, p. 1366–1367.
3. Grafstrom, R. & Curren, R. "Genotoxicity of formaldehyde in cultured human bronchial fibroblasts." *Science,* 1985, 228: 89–90.
4. Sittig, M. *Handbook of Toxic and Hazardous Chemicals and Carcinogens,* pp. 868–869.
5. Beebe, G. *Toxic Carpet III.* Cincinnati, Ohio: Beebe, 1991, pp. 138–237.
6. Brodeur, P. *The Great Power Line Coverup.* New York: Little, Brown & Company, 1993.
7. Breysse, P. "ELF magnetic field exposures in an office environment." *American Journal of Industrial Medicine,* 1994, 25: 177–185.
8. Sittig, M. *Handbook of Hazardous Chemicals and Carcinogens,* pp. 29, 931.

45. Safe? Who's Kidding Who?

1. Bergin, E. & Grandon, R. *How to Survive in Your Toxic Environment.* New York: Avon Books, 1984.
2. National Research Council. *Toxicity Testing: Strategies to Determine Needs and Priorities,* Washington, D.C.: National Academy Press, 1984.
3. Duggan, R. "Dietary intake of pesticide chemicals in the United States." *Pesticides Monitoring Journal,* 1968, 2: 140–152.
4. *Mainstream,* summer 1983, 17.
5. "The EPA and regulation of pesticides." Staff report to the Subcommittee on Administrative Practice and Procedure." Washington, D.C.: United States Senate, 1974, p. 24.

ES

6. Regenstein, L. *How To Survive in America the Poisoned.* New York: Acropolis Books, 1982, p. 368.

7. Butler, W. & Warren, J. "Petition for suspension and cancellation of chlordane/heptachlor." Washington, D.C.: Environmental Defense Fund, 1974.

8. "The EPA and the Regulation of Pesticides." Staff report to Subcommittee on Administrative Practice and Procedure, U.S. Senate, Dec. 1976, p. 7556.

9. Paddock, R. "Chemical ok'd for farms despite safety questions." *Los Angeles Times,* May 31, 1991, A28.

10. Diem, G. "Threshold limit values—how good are they?" *Environmental Health News,* 1991, 7–9.

11. Van Strum, C. & Merrell, P. "Dioxin human health damage studies: damaged data?" *Journal of Pesticide Reform,* 1990, 10(1): 8.

12. Regenstein, L. *How To Survive in America the Poisoned.* New York: Acropolis Books, 1982.

13. See note 1 above.

14. Russell, D. "The rise of the grass-roots toxic movement." *Amicus Journal,* 1990, 18–21.

15. Natural Resources Defense Council. *Twenty-Five-Year Report (1970–1995).* New York: Natural Resources Defense Council, 1995, pp. 1–15.

16. See note 1 above.

46. You Can Have It, I Don't Want It

1. "Exporting banned and hazardous pesticides." *FASE Reports.* Los Angeles: The Foundation for Advancements in Science and Education, 1991, 9(1): 1–6.

2. Scanlan, C. "America's killer exports." *San Jose Mercury News,* May 19, 1991.

3. McConnell, R. & Hruska, A. "An epidemic of pesticide poisoning in Nicaragua: implications for prevention in developing countries." *American Journal of Public Health,* 1993, 83(11): 1559–1562.

4. Jeyaratnam, J. "Acute pesticide poisoning: a major global health problem." *World Health Statistics Quarterly,* 1990, 43(3): 139–144.

5. Jeyaratnam, J. "Health problems of pesticide usage in the third world." *British Journal of Industrial Medicine,* 1985, 42: 505–506.

6. Steele, I. *Development Forum,* 1990.

7. "Exporting banned and hazardous pesticides: a preliminary report." *FASE Reports.* Los Angeles: The Foundation for Advancements in Science and Education, 1991, 9(1): S-2.

8. See note 4 above.

9. Steinman, D. & Epstein, S.S. *The Safe Shopper's Bible.* New York: Macmillan, 1995, pp. 317, 325.

10. See note 7 above.

47. A Man Named Delaney

1. Ames, B., et al. "Rodent carcinogens: setting priorities." *Science,* 1993, 258: 261–265.

2. Davis, D., et al. "International trends in cancer mortality in France, West Germany, Italy, Japan, England and Wales, and the USA." *The Lancet,* 1990: 475–480.

3. Pimentel, D., et al. "An assessment of the environmental and economic impacts of pesticide use." In: Briggs, S.A. and Rachel Carson Council. *Basic Guide to Pesticides.* Washington, D.C.: Hemisphere Publishing, 1992.

4. Hansen, M. *Escape From the Pesticide Treadmill.* Mount Vernon, N.Y.: Institute for Consumer Policy Research: Consumers Union, 1987.

5. "Court cramps EPA on pesticides." *Science,* 1992, 257: 322.

6. "U.S. Appeals Court upholds Delaney clause; strikes down EPA decision to allow four carcinogenic pesticides in processed food." *National Coalition Against the Misuse of Pesticides: Technical Report,* 1992, 7(8): 1–4.

48. Follow the Money

1. Stauber, J. *PR Watch.*

2. Meadows, D. "Freedom of disinformation." *The Amicus Journal,* Fall 1991, 11.

3. Hawken, P. *The Ecology of Commerce.* New York: HarperCollins, 1993, p. 129.

4. See note 2 above.

5. Hawken, P. *The Ecology of Commerce,* pp. 178–179.

6. Epstein, S.S. "Needless new risk of breast cancer." *Los Angeles Times,* March 20, 1994: M5.

7. Schneider, K. "Congressmen seek inquiry of milk-hormone approval." *The New York Times,* April 18, 1994: A8

8. Epstein, S.S. "Polluted data." *The Sciences,* New York Academy of Sciences, July/August 1978, 16–21.

9. Epstein, S.S. *The Politics of Cancer.* San Francisco: Sierra Club Books, 1978, p. 301.

49. Rock the Vote

1. Anonymous. "100-day national environmental scorecard details Congress's negative actions on conservation issues." Press Release, April 18, 1995. Washington, D.C.: League of Conservation Voters.

2. Ibid.

3. Ibid.

4. Hawken, P. *The Ecology of Commerce,* New York: Harper Collins, 1993, p. 177.

5. Ibid., p. 183.

50. Throw the Book at It!

1. Henley, D. & Marsh, D. *Heaven Is Under Our Feet,* Stamford, Conn.: Longmeadow Press, 1991, pp. 102–108.